The Male S

The Survival Arsenal

"A true warrior only fights the
battle he can win."
(Sun Tze, The Art of War)

"Know your enemy well and in a
100 battles, you will merge
victoriously."
(Sun Tze, The Art of War)

The Male Sexual Warrior

Copyright © 2017 by Dr. Angelo Isom, ND, CHS, MQT

Visit my website for future updates, products and services. Phone consults are available via appointments as well.

ISBN-13: 978-1547069668

www.lifeishealing.com

www.harmonizingfist.com

Medical Disclaimer

The information provided in this book is designed to provide helpful information on the subjects discussed. This book is not meant to be used, nor should it be used, to diagnose or treat any medical condition. For diagnosis or treatment of any medical problem, consult your own physician. The publisher and author are not responsible for any specific health or allergy needs that may require medical supervision and are not liable for any damages or negative consequences from any treatment, action, application or preparation, to any person reading or following the information in this book. References are provided for informational purposes only.

Brief Biography of Dr. Angelo Isom, ND, CHS, MQT

Dr. Angelo Isom is a graduate of New York University, Columbia University, Georgia State University and Clayton College of Natural Healing. He holds several degrees in various fields including psychology, philosophy, teaching methods, education and naturopathy and numerous other certifications. He is a male health advisor, martial arts lineage holder and researcher.

Dr. Isom's experiences in healing encompass multiple areas of research and study. Some of these areas include acupuncture, yoga, internal martial arts, qi gong, energy healing, human sexuality, western and eastern herbs, diet and nutrition. Dr. Isom is the author of several books and video available on lifeishealing.com. This list includes:

The Sexual Warrior Within

Are You Healthy for Sex?

Life Is Healing Qigong

The 5 Yin Organs Taoist Medical Qigong (DVD)

Dr. Isom has been fortunate to study cultural healing methods and herbs while visiting such countries as Brazil, Mexico's Yucatan Peninsula, Panama, Haiti,

Jamaica and Puerto Rico. Dr. Isom is CEO and Director of Life is Healing, a holistic wellness ministry.

Over the years, he has counseled many clients seeking to achieve optimal fitness and health and has appeared as a guest speaker in workshops and health expos.

Dr. Isom's approach to healing and rejuvenation focuses upon the cultivation of vital energy of qi, grounding, internal cleansing, eating according to the seasons, mind/body balance, and lifestyle.

For more information visit:
www.lifeishealing.com
www.harmonizingfist.com

Reviews

"Dr. Isom has done an excellent job in showcasing sexual issues that plaque men of all ages today. Men can now feel optimistic in choosing a solution that is right for them. I highly recommend that every man young and old read the Sexual Warrior Within. Women should definitely buy this book for their lover or husband"
---- C. Blackburn, Health and Wellness Coach

"Finally, man's modern day natural guide for herbal Viagra without the side effects. Read and study this book and you will be on the right track."
---- C. Parks, Nurse LPN and Holistic Healing Counselor and Advocate.

"After following Dr. Isom's teachings on qi gong and taking natural herbs I have experienced more skeletal flexibility and internal organ strength. The information in the Sexual Warrior Within has improved my health, sex life, and mental attitude."
David T. --- retired railroad worker and robust 65 year young.

"Being a media professional is demanding both physically and mentally. I began a health regimen of internal martial arts, qigong, and herbal supplements under Dr. Isom. My health has improved since I began, I am better able to focus and work at my best level."
 - --**Tau Justice, Southside Media, LLC.**

"It is easy to tell that Dr. Isom is very passionate about this subject. He has dedicated a great deal of his life to help men regain their confidence and sense of manhood. With this book, men will not only have the knowledge of what to do if they are having various male issues, but they will also have the power to prevent these issues in the first place. I am very excited about the knowledge that Dr. Isom has brought forth. This book is really a game changer." --- **Crystal Lawrence, MBA**

"This book is a must read for both men and women. For men, it is a handbook for healthy living and sexual vitality. With this tool, men will no longer be dependent upon sexual wellness or stamina drugs. Dr. Isom's book provides freedom of choice. Stamina and endurance can be achieved naturally free of drugs without damaging side effects. Every woman that has a man in her life should also be knowledgeable about the options presented to men through this book.

Women are key motivators to their mates; and in return, can encourage their partners to follow the lifestyle changes that are presented. In summary, this is everyone's book." **ChieStine Lawrence, Computer Technology Engineer, IT Consultant.**

Preface

This book was developed out of the need to consolidate my personal research and insightful discoveries about human sexuality and performance issues often encountered by men. Many of my notes were often scattered across my work desk either buried in old folders, internet files or simply lost due to my failure to document properly. One day, I thought wouldn't it be great if most of my research could be consolidated in one reliable sustainable place. It was then that I decided on placing them into a book format for retrieval. Getting started and organizing information seemed to be quite intimidating for someone like me that usually post information anywhere for convenience. After hours, days and weeks of cleaning up, evaluating and reorganizing mounds of information and data, I reconstructed my archive. The next big step was outlining and updating my research with current research.

Gradually everything became clear and I began to process my notes in a systematic concise way. Imposing discipline upon myself to write daily turned out to be one of several the key factors for my success. After 6 months of continuous writing I still had to overcome numerous problems with editing, copywriting, ISBN and marketing. In the end, the final path was made clear and worth the journey.

Dedication

This book is dedicated to all the members of my immediate and extended family for their kindness, inspiration and devotion. I would like to extend special thanks to all of my martial arts students, family and friends, especially Eric Graham, Tau Justice for there support in convincing me that I should write this book and have it published. Special thanks to Crystal and ChieStine Lawrence for assisting me in the promotion of my book by creating the lifeishealing.com website and for their dedication and support of my business endeavors. Last but not least, an enduring thanks to Cathy Blackburn for her support on the design of the book cover. This book is also dedicated to all men who struggle day to day to be the man that they were meant to be. All men who want to preserve their health and maintain healthy testosterone levels should read and study this book. A healthy sex life is well worth pursuing. Many men struggle quietly every day to be healthy, loving, romantic and sexy but often encounter many obstacles. Settling for impotency or being celibate is not an option or forced choice.

The sexual warrior within each man does not want to lay down arms and surrender to the emasculating process of modern living. Some men simply accepted defeat or allowed themselves to become easily disillusioned.

It is my goal to recruit them once again and harness the sexual warrior within. It is my goal that the reader will greatly benefit from the knowledge and practical strategies given in this book to preserve and recover their sexual lifestyle.

Table of Contents

The Mind / Body Connection/Affirmations

Many men tend to overlook the importance of the mind body connection when it comes to sex. Sex is not all physical in nature. This connection can have profound influence on a man's health, vitality and erectile power. Using positive affirmation daily can rewire your mental habits and subconscious beliefs can influence the biological processes of the entire body.

By regularly conditioning your mind with these affirmations you will encourage your body to send blood flow to your penis, strengthen the tissue and muscle in the pelvis, and naturally increase your sex drive. Thoughts are everything. The way we think empowers our daily actions and health. Thoughts can affect hormonal balance shifting us into high or low gear. When the word is spoken, it is materialized as intent leading us to a specific course of action and outcome.

I encourage you not to underestimate the power of affirmations. When saying affirmations, one must match the proper emotional element with it. Emotional content combine with a directive affirmation leads to personal manifested power.

Affirmations without an emotional root are impotent. Review the following affirmations and decide which of them is applicable. Choose well.

"Change your thoughts and you change the world"
- Norman Vincent Peale

AFFIRMATIONS FOR SEXUAL POWER

Present Tense Affirmations
I am sexually confident
I am a great lover
I am a powerful sexual being
I am in touch with my deepest sexual nature and desire
I always please my partner
I am open to new sexual experiences
I am secure in my body and celebrate its sexuality
I express my deepest sexual needs
I am a sexually confident man
My penis is strong and hard
My body directs blood flow to my penis
My penis has excellent circulation
My erections are long lasting
My partner is turned on by my hardness
I am free from worry and stress
I am revitalizing my penile tissue with the power of my mind
I always achieve erection
My penis is healthy

Future Tense Affirmations
I will unleash my sexual confidence
I will express my sexual nature
I am developing magnetic sexual power
I am becoming sexually confident
My sexual confidence is growing
I am overcoming my sexual insecurities
I am starting to explore my wildest fantasies
I will provide immense sexual pleasure to my partner
I am becoming a highly skilled lover
I am noticing my partner is turned on by my sexual confidence

My Personal Quotes and Thoughts

Sex is only good as it is leveraged.

All men have the right to life, liberty and the pursuit of sex.

Men must say no to celibacy and yes to orgasm.

Next to life itself sex is the one of the greatest gifts in the world.

Men are at risk today and tomorrow when it comes to a healthy a sex life. Sex can not be taken for granted.

The notion of manhood is constantly being redefined.

The world is becoming more feminine everyday.

Having a normal testosterone level is considered an endangered event.

Your life is your sex and sex is your life.

Without dopamine, there is no lust. Without lust, there is no sex.

Men with low testosterone levels are easy to control and manipulate.

"Live Your Life by Design and Not Fate"

You only miss 100% of the women you don't pursue and the conquest you leave to fate.

Every man is a sexual warrior.

Being sexually active is a good index of health

Without strong male sexual energy, a nation cannot secure its future and survive upheavals.

The right of passage to manhood has been deleted from our culture and is no longer treated as a right.

I am the lord and master of my bedroom.

Keep sex alive!

> "Instead of focusing on the woman you want try focusing your time and energy on the woman that wants you."

Don't be a man that needs a woman but rather the man that a woman needs.

Homo-sapien equals <u>Homo-erectus</u> from a sexual point of view.

Without life there is no sex.
Without sex there is no life.

All Men Should Strive to Become an Alpha Male = I (AM)

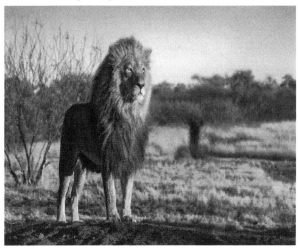

Being an alpha male, (AM) has more to do with attitude than altitude or size. Simply put it's all about empowerment. An AM leads, direct, controls while achieving dominance over his dominion and sexual lifestyle. He utilizes all of his resources and dedicates himself to being 100% of the man he can be. The AM sets the standard for his right to passage into manhood. Most women are conditioned to desire, respect and fantasize about being ravished by a gentle AM. He literally tends to dominate the bedroom. Many women are taught to settle for an omega male, (OM) out of need or in exchange for modern day financial security. The OM is conditioned to lose, settle and be easily dominated by both men and other women. Men that are controlled by their wives are omega males.

Women in general are usually empathetic and tolerant of a man's shortcomings. Because of their enormous capacity for compassion and love, women tolerate an OM if he makes a commitment to care for her, raise and protect the family. Given this scenario and the pressures of social obligations, the notion of prioritizing a healthy sex life is usually reduced to the status of a secondary fantasy.

An AM can be defined as a winner who takes what he wants, maintains his conquest while being willing to pay the price to do so. Many of the world's formidable Alpha Males were also bold daring men of small physical stature. Some examples of these men, to name a few, could include Napoleon, Bruce Lee, and Geronimo.

Introduction

This book was written as a non-technical guide with detailed explanation to help the reader better understand why and how the male sexual energy system works. Once understood, the reader will be better able to apply more appropriate strategies and interventions to help restore sexual vitality. Sexual energy manifests itself in more ways than just the all too familiar romantic interplay between man and woman or lust. It is by nature the creative potential energy that drives the artist, boxer or entrepreneur. Sexual energy can manifest itself as the source of courage and commitment needed to start a new business or investment in a risky but profitable business venture. Simply put, it is the motivation and raw desire to succeed at a given task or goal leading to a more pleasurable outcome. All great men and leaders throughout history shared a common thread of heighten primal sexual energy transformed or transmuted into a specific goal. This is why, it is vital for all people to cultivate, preserve and protect their sexual energy. Our sexual energy can also have a profound impact on our daily health.

Many studies have shown that sexual energy and health are often correlated.

The key ingredients are often indicative of a good heart and robust circulation of blood and hormones.

Without health, there is no sex. Without sex health does not thrive. Good sexual energy can save marriages, boost our immune system, improve prostate health, regulating a woman's menstrual cycle and sometimes even prevent wars.

It is my quest to sexually empower the average male by increasing awareness to multicultural and global alternatives integrated with modern wisdom. I commend those men who still want to engage in vigorous sexual activity but feel compromised by lack of health and poor lifestyle choices.

If you want to get your body and your sex life back on track, you'll find the tools and strategies you need to make it happen right here.

Many men fail to understand that there are indeed a plethora of solutions that are natural and noninvasive waiting to be discovered. Viagra free erections are still a reality worth pursing. The average male no longer needs to rely exclusively upon drugs such as Viagra and synthetic low testosterone gels highly publicized on TV commercials, radio and magazines. During ancient times if a warrior dropped his sword he could easily lose his life. The sword symbolized the warrior's manhood, ability to fight and preserve his freedom and sexual potency. Today the stakes are quite similar for modern man.

The sword is now symbolic modern man's his genital and sexual potency.

Be aware that there are always constant threats looming in the background that can threaten one's manhood. If the sexual warrior drops his testosterone level and libido too low then he too could lose his sex life.

All warriors should have an attitude of readiness and resolve to win and or survive any confrontation. A healthy sex life is worth fighting for. The sexual warrior should be dedicated to maintaining a healthy readiness status to engage in the art of lovemaking when ever confronted by a beautiful consensual woman.

It is nature and inner nature that will guide each man down the right path without risks of dangerous side effects and dependency upon synthetic aphrodisiacs. Many men simply do not realize that there is a daily ongoing battle raging within themselves trying to find that delicate balance of hormones, libido and erection power. Proper peripheral blood flow and testosterone levels can fluctuate from moment to moment and day-to-day.

Every metabolic process in the body must be timed correctly. The hormonal or endocrine system of the body can be compared to a car.

If the engine of a car is not tuned or timed properly, it will fail to crank or maintain combustion.

Quite similar to the human body many of these internal processes are time sensitive. A more detailed explanation of these biochemical processes will be discussed later in the chapter on the Biology of Libido.

After much research on sexual energy, personal exploration and surveying of numerous personal testimonies, I became compelled to write this book. The gradual decline of both libido and sexual vigor should not be understood as a natural process of aging. This belief model is far from the truth especially when we compare modern man to the indigenous tribal communities of Latin America, Africa and Native Americans. These people are far healthier and robust in terms of fertility, libido and sexual energy. What are their secrets? How are these people able to remain in hormonal paradise? Many of these people live in close alliance with nature and continue to maintain sexual vigor well into their 90s.

Many ancient healing and sexual enhancement practices are often misunderstood or tabooed. The dawning of a new sexual revolution and renaissance that fosters enhancement, performance and true intimacy awaits the reader of this book. The science of present day knowledge and its modus operandi for improving male sexual potency is also analyzed in detail with regards to pros and cons. Men everywhere should no longer have to resort to sacrificing long term health for short term gains using conventional means. What we need today is a paradigm shift of thinking. This new model of thinking states that one can be physically fit at any age and be sexually active as well. Issues relating to sexual problems must be attacked from many angles using a variety of approaches such as testosterone supplements, ejaculation control, chemical avoidance, and estrogen reduction etc.

Chapter 1

Age Related Sexual Decline in Male Sexual Performance

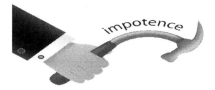

Sexual performance is probably the most common concern of both young and aging men as it relates to their health and relationships. The average man's sexual peak usually occurs around the age of 18. Due to poor diet and the stresses of modern living and unhealthy lifestyles significant declines in sexual performances can occur as early as 26 years of age. Most men began to notice a longer time needed to be aroused and to achieve a full erection. These problems can range from a less than firm erection, lower libido, decrease in sexual stamina and lower volume of ejaculation during orgasm.

As men age, there is usually a drop in the production of hormones such as DHEA, testosterone and other related androgens or sex hormones. When men reach the age of 40 their testosterone level can decrease by 1% for each following year. Research clearly shows that about 20% of men in their 60s and 50% of men in their 80's have significantly reduced testosterone levels.

As testosterone is a key hormone in men's sexual function, aging-related decline in testosterone levels can have a negative impact on self-esteem and sexual performance.

As sexual performance is closely related to men's overall health, factors that affect general health, such as anxiety, stress, and psychological factors, can also affect sexual performance. Fortunately, any decline associated with these factors can usually be reversed once the underlying causes are resolved.

There is a light at the end of this tunnel. Many of these symptoms of decline that are age-related can actually be reversed. What is most important and part of the solution is having a stress-free and active healthy lifestyle. Many men notice a distinct improvement in sexual performance and overall health when smoking, alcohol and recreational drug use are eliminated or kept to a minimum.

Low testosterone level can be medically treated by testosterone replacement therapy. The goal of this therapy is to increase serum levels of testosterone by means of injection, oral dosage and trans-dermal delivery of testosterone.

Testosterone replacement therapy can also be risky if one chooses this approach.

Close monitoring of serum androgen levels should be done periodically by a qualified physician.

The use of herbal extracts and formulations have clinically been shown to offer a more promising solution in reversing age-related decline in men.

Protodiocin is one of the active compounds found an herbal plant commonly known as Tribulus Terrestris. Tribulus clinically has been shown the ability to increase both the level of DHEA and testosterone in men.

One clinical study on 15 men with decreased sexual performance indicated that nearly 90% of them treated with Tribulus at 500 mg 3X daily for 60 days experience a significantly improved libido, ejaculation, and orgasm as compared to before the treatment.

Protodioscin treatment resulted in significantly increased sex drive 33% of men after 30 days and in 80% of men after 60 days. Similarly, arousal improved in 53% of men after 30 days and 87% of men after 60 days. Orgasm sensation and ejaculate quality also improved significantly in 40% and 87% of men after 30 and 60 days.

In another clinical study, 60 non-diabetic men with and without erectile dysfunctions and 15 diabetic men with sexual performance problems were given protodioscin) at 3 x 250 mg per day for 3 weeks.

The study found that in addition to increased DHEA levels in the treated group, the frequency of successful intercourse increased by 60%. In addition, an improved sense of well-being, improved sensation, erection, ejaculation, and orgasm were also reported by the treated men. In these and other clinical studies on Tribulus protodioscin, there were no unwanted side effects or contraindications.

Tribulus Terrestris is slowly becoming a very popular herb. Unfortunately, not all commercially available Tribulus contain the active ingredient protodioscin at the standardized level or dosage to produce results. A saponin level of 45% or higher is needed by most men to duplicate the same level of success as seen in the research studies.

References:

1. Morley, JE. Testosterone replacement in older men and women. J Gend Specif Med. 2001; 4:49-53

2. Viktorov I, Bozadjieva E, Protich M, et al. Pharmacological, pharmacokinetic, toxicological and clinical studies on protodioscin. 1994, IIMS Therapeutic Focus

3. Arsyad KM. Effect of protodioscin on the quantity and quality of sperms from males with moderate idiopathic oligozoospermia. Medika 22 (8): 614-618 (1996)

4. Adimoelja A and Ganeshan Adaikan P. Protodioscin from herbal plant Tribulus terrestris L improves the male sexual functions, probably via DHEA. Int. J. Impotence Research. 1997:9; Supp. 1

Chapter 2

Are You Healthy Enough to Have Sex?

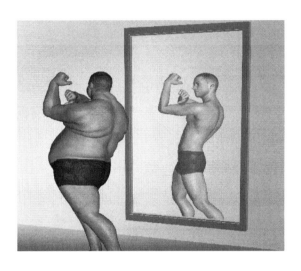

How healthy and physically fit are you? One should strive to be physically fit at any age. Many men tend to ignore the fact that having sex can be a very physically demanding act. During a typical erotic encounter, there are dramatic physical changes that occurs n the body and brain. Both respiration and heart rate are normally elevated in anticipation along with increase in blood pressure. These bodily reactions are quite similar to what athletes experience just prior to competition or warm-ups. Other common reactions can also include muscle tension, perspiration, release of pheromones, nervousness, elevated stress hormones like cortisol, an increase of adrenaline and of course the release of testosterone. Some of these physical changes are conducive for good sex and some of them can get in the way. Most athletes are very familiar with performance anxiety which can impair their ability.

My new paradigm shift of thinking advocates that men should train for sex. Most people clearly recognize that in order to be good at sports you must train or workout on a regular basis. The physical training must fit the specific physical requirement of the sport. Why not do the same for sex? The term often used by coaches is called "Specificity of Training".

You may be surprised to learn what the simple definition of physical fitness. Physical Fitness is a measure of the body's ability to function efficiently and effectively in work and leisure activities, resist hypo-kinetic diseases (diseases from sedentary lifestyles), and to meet emergency situations. This definition was derived from decades of research by exercise physiologists and cardiologists.

The top 10 facets of physical fitness are adapted from sources that include the President Council on Fitness, Sports & Nutrition, Cross Fit, and the National Strength & Conditioning Association.

Physical Fitness # 1 **Body Composition**

Definition: The relative amount of fat, muscle, bone, and other vital parts of the body.

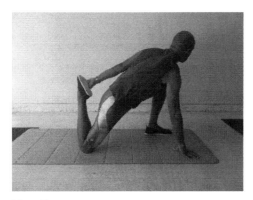

Dr. Isom

Measurement: Skin fold calipers, BIA, DEXA (see ways to measure body fat percentage)

Body Composition is always important. It is possible for an individual to have a high degree of fitness and still have excess body fat. Losing body fat while retaining lean muscle mass will improve all other physical attributes. Strength/power to weight ratio will also be improved along with other general health markers.

Physical Fitness # 2- **Strength**

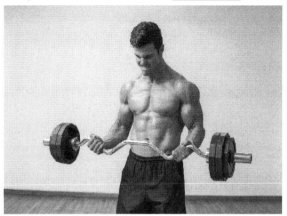

Strength is required to perform basic functional movements in our life like squatting, lunging, pushing, pulling, and bending are important in our everyday life. In addition, as we age muscle size and strength tend to decrease along with bone mass, which can be reversed with strength training. Measurement: Multiple tests must be completed to test more than one muscle group. Examples include max effort on exercises like the squat, bench press, or dead lift from 1-6 repetitions.

Physical Fitness #3 | **Cardiovascular Fitness**

Definition: Ability of the circulatory systems and respiratory systems to supply oxygen during sustained physical activity.

Measurement: VO2 Max Test, sub-maximal YMCA

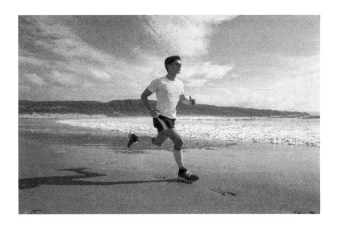

Significance: Cardiovascular exercises increase lung capacity so the heart does not have to work as hard to pump blood to the muscles. Respiration is important for overall heart health and prevention of lifestyle diseases.

Definition: Ability of the circulatory systems and respiratory systems to supply oxygen during sustained physical activity.

Measurement: VO2 Max Test, sub-maximal YMCA Step Test

Significance: An improved cardiovascular system increases lung capacity so the heart does not have to work as hard.

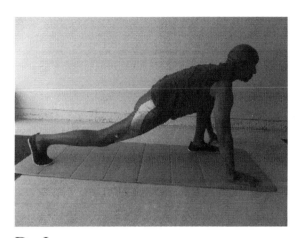

Dr. Isom

Physical Fitness #4 | **Flexibility**

Definition: The range of motion at a joint

Measurement: There is no specific test because there are many joints in the human body, but a range of stretches can identify flexibility like the sit and reach test, shoulder reach etc. Significance: The optimal range of motion about various joints has a direct effect on almost all other facets of physical fitness. For example, if one's hip flexors are tight, that can affect the ability to reach maximum speed, or perform agility drills at a high level. For some flexibility is innate while others have to work hard to acquire it. Flexibility should always be approached gradually without strain and pain.

A realistic expectation of improving one's range of motion should be based upon correct stretching method, consistent routines and warm-ups.

Physical Fitness #5 | **Muscular Endurance**

Definition: The ability of muscles to continue to perform repeated contractions.

Measurement: Given there is more than one major muscle group, testing muscular endurance requires testing each individual muscle, or group. Examples include maximum number of push-ups, sit-ups, pull-ups, and dips.

Significance: Performing repetitious physical activity such as gardening, raking leaves and washing your car are common activities that can improve endurance.

Health, Nutrition, and Wellness – Mental fitness, nutrition and wellness are also integral parts of optimal fitness. In fact, optimal fitness could never be achieved without adequate mental fitness and proper nutrition.

One should clearly understand why physical fitness is so important when it comes to being able to have good sex. Top priority should be given to fitness before considering the use of Viagra/Cialis or Low T topical gels to boost overall wellness and libido.

Do you have back pains and bad knees?

Well according to Chinese medicine these are symptoms of what is called unbalanced kidney qi (energy). The concept of qi is becoming more common in the west today. Every function of one's body requires sustained energy. There are herbal formulations and special exercises which will be discussed later to help balance the qi levels in the body. Having low back pains and knee problems can really interfere with our ability to have and enjoy sex.

How does blood circulation affect my sex life?

In order to achieve an erection, blood must be able to flow to the peripheral area of our bodies such as the penis. If circulation is impaired by any arterial diseases or high blood pressure medication, a man will not be able to achieve or sustain an erection. Exercise in general is one of the best cures for enhancing blood circulation to all areas of the body. Stress on the other hand, can constrict blood vessels and significantly reduce their flow. An all natural vasodilator such as gingko biloba and nervine herb such as passion flower can be very helpful in remedying this problem.

Am I emotionally or mentally balanced?
Sexual activity should be a positive and pleasant experience between two consensual people.

Sex can also cause men to experience negative emotions such as disappointment, anxiety, humiliation and frustration and even rage. This can easily happen if men feel that the quality and standards of sex they seek is not possible. Impotency and anguish are often the result. All men should learn to forgive themselves and strive to correct these problems rather than worrying about them.

What are 3 most common diseases that can impairs sex directly or indirectly?
If you guess correctly, they are heart disease, diabetes and hypertension. These diseases can incapacitate a man's performance directly or due to the side effects of medication. These diseases must be kept under proper control while one is seeking a life style change leading to a more permanent cure.

Do you sleep 6-8 hours per night?

Lack of adequate REM sleep can cause many of our hormones to be out of balance.

All the sex pills in the world can not compare to the rejuvenating effect of a good night sleep. Night sleep rebalances and promotes healthy hormone levels especially testosterone.

Our bodies heal itself by regenerating cells and organs restoring us to a more helpful balance. Pushing our bodies beyond our energy reserve will inevitably weaken our bodies triggering our immune system to go into overdrive. Our immune system consumes huge volumes of energy balancing itself daily. Without a good night of sleep, one can only expect a lower threshold of energy for sex. Sexual vitality works best when there is a surplus or reserve energy or qi in the body.

Do you drink excessively?

A small amount of alcohol can be beneficial for sex. A small amount of alcohol can actually dilate and relax blood vessels resulting in increase blood flow to the penis and internal organs. In contrast, excessive consumption of alcohol can literally turn off the pilot light of vitality. Even moderate alcohol consumption tends to decrease the vital sex nutrient, zinc.

Keep in mind, that zinc is a necessary precursor for the production of testosterone.

Excess alcohol will impair or slow down the necessary vitality and adrenaline we need to have sex. No man wants to go to sleep on the job of making love.

Are you a smoker?

Smoking is definitely out of the question. Smoking is equally bad due to the depletion of oxygen in the body. Lack of oxygen can rob the blood cells of energy and reduce flow to the sex organs.

When oxygen levels are reduced to the brain by excess smoking the quality and volume of blood flow to the penis will also diminish. A man's breathing capacity may very well be an index of his potential strength and sexual endurance. Without proper breathing a man can not control his ejaculation or erectile strength. The breath of life must be respected and cultivated. Where there is breath there is life. The livelier a man is the deeper he breathes and the more sexual vitality is at his command.

References:

Marc Perry, CSCS, CPT | February 21, 2012 | Updated:
June 4, 2013
JAMA and Archives Journals. "Fitness Level, Not Body
Fat, May Be Stronger Predictor Of Longevity For Older
Adults." ScienceDaily. ScienceDaily, 5 December 2007.
<www.sciencedaily.com/releases/2007/12/07120416324
9.htm>.
Kaptchuk, TedChinese Medicine, The Web That has no
Weaver Rider, London, 1983 (Kidney Qi
Mirone V, Ricci E, Gentile V, Basile Fasolo C, Parazzini
F. Determinants of erectile dysfunction risk in a large
series of Italian men attending andrology clinics. Eur
Urol. 2004;45:87–91. [PubMed]

4. The Way of the Herb, Michael Tierra, 1998 Pocket
books, Gingko p. 139-140.

5. Van Thiel DH, Lester R. The effect of chronic alcohol
abuse on sexual function. th Clin Endocrinol Metab.
1979;8:499–510. [PubMed]

6. Jensen SB, Gludd C. Sexual dysfunction in men with
alcoholic liver cirrhosis: A comparative study. Liver.

1985;5:94–100. [PubMed]

7. Mirone V, Ricci E, Gentile V, Basile Fasolo C, Parazzini F. Determinants of erectile dysfunction risk in a large series of Italian men attending andrology clinics. Eur Urol. 2004;45:87–91. [PubMed]

8. Van Thiel DH, Lester R. The effect of chronic alcohol abuse on sexual function. th Clin Endocrinol Metab. 1979;8:499–510. [PubMed]

9. Jensen SB, Gludd C. Sexual dysfunction in men with alcoholic liver cirrhosis: A comparative study. Liver. 1985;5:94–100. [PubMed]

Chapter 3

The Biology and Chemistry of Libido Simplified

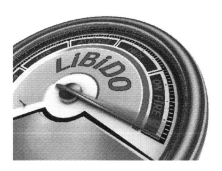

The biology and chemistry of sex is sometimes difficult to fathom for the average non- medical layman. There are numerous bio-chemical processes involving enzymes, hormones, vasodilators and neural brain transmitters all working in sync with each other at the right time to make one's libido and sex life functional.

Many men often ask why is it necessary to understand these underlying processes in order to have a healthy sex life. The answer is often simple. What you don't know can harm or hinder your potential. In terms of problems related to sex, you can't fix something if you don't know what needs to be fixed.

Impotency or lack of sex drive can be symptomatic of many health problems and must be addressed in an individualized manner.

The one pill fits all approach certainly does not work for everyone. Viagra or Cialis should not be the first step taken when things are not going well in the bedroom most men tend to look for a quick fix rather than a long-term solution.

A quick fix will not withstand the test of time nor is it necessarily good for one's health. Men should not opt to jeopardize their overall long-term health for the momentary delight of a sexual encounter. I am sure many of us have heard the argument, if I am going to die, then I rather die having sex, as justification to taking steroids, synthetic testosterone and overdosing on sex pills.

Here's a quick test. *

What is the most important organ in the body that having good sex depends upon the most? Pause!

The answer is the brain. Sexual arousal starts in the mind by way of perception or anticipation of an erotic event. If your body and mind are not working in harmony, you will not be able to perform as you desire. Engaging in a sexual act requires mental focus as well as physical energy.

Let us begin our lesson with defining a few simple terms such as hormone, enzyme, vasodilator and a brain neurotransmitter.

Hormones are biochemical messengers that are released from glands in the body to trigger specific physical processes such as the release testosterone, adrenaline and estrogen to name a few.

They also tend to bind to receptor sites in the body where they are needed.

Enzymes are biochemical compounds that speed up or enable certain reactions to occur. An example of this is aromatase which triggers the unfortunate conversion of free flowing testosterone into estrogen. Vasodilators refer to a class of substances that can expand or open up a blood vessel and increase its flow. Aspirin is a common example.

Brain Neurotransmitters are brain chemicals like hormones that can turn on or off specific reactions in the body. A good example of this compound is the euphoric blissful bonding experienced following an orgasm due to the release of oxytocin and endorphins. The love hormone, oxytocin is known to be plentiful in lactating women and is released by both men and women after an orgasm.

What causes an erection?

Erection of the penis is one of the most important physiological processes to occur in males regardless of their age, genetic make-up or geographic location. Most men usually associate the erection of the penis with sexual arousal. This is not necessary true. Erections can occur on a regular basis without the premeditated thought of a sexual arousing image or event. The average healthy male can have 4-8 erections at night while sleeping and dreaming. There are 3 distinct stages of penile erection.

Arousal: The man becomes sexually aroused via thought and association.

Erection: The penis responds by becoming erect and firm.

Ejaculation: Physical stimulation of the penis causes the release of semen.

If, by any chance, step two (erection) does not happen, step three (ejaculation) becomes difficult or almost impossible. This condition can lead to what is called "male impotence".

What is the role of the brain in causing an erection?

The penis is one of the places in the body where the brain needs to be able to turn the blood flow on and off with a thought. When a man is sexually stimulated by sight, thought, or touch, the brain sends signals that relax the smooth muscles around the arteries that supply blood to the corpora cavernosa. The veins draining the blood cannot keep up, resulting in swelling. As the swelling reaches the limit of the penile skin, the penis becomes firm.

The pressure of the spongy corpora cavernosa against the skin partially closes the veins, helping to maintain the erection. Erection continues until the signals from the brain stop, but erections are seldom consistent. Waxing and waning like the moon are normal responses even during intercourse.

What is the role of the corpora cavernosa?

The penis uses a similar mechanism, but instead of using pressurized air to become rigid, the penis uses pressurized blood. The penis contains two cigar-shaped structures, called corpora cavernosa (singular: corpus cavernosum), that it uses to become erect. You can think of the corpora cavernosa as balloon-like tubes. Arteries bring blood into these two tubes and veins carry blood away from them. The corpora cavernosa expandS to hold 90% of the blood involved in an erection, increasing both in length and in diameter. The function of the corpus spongiosum is to prevent compression of the urethra during erection.The penis can be either limp or erect, depending on the flow of blood. Inside the shaft of the penis are three columns of erectile tissue—the two corpora cavernosa, which run parallel to each other along the top of the penis, and the corpus spongiosum, which runs along the bottom of the penis and surrounds the urethra.

Despite the fact that erections are often called "boners," there are no bones within the penis. During an erection, the corpora cavernosa and the corpus spongiosum, which are rich in blood vessels become engorged with blood. This expansion makes the penis larger and firmer. The fancy name for this is "vaso-congestion."

In a non-erect state, the arteries that bring blood into the corpora cavernosa are somewhat constricted, while the veins that drain the blood from the penis are open.
There is no way for pressure to build inside the penis. In this state, the penis is limp. When a man becomes aroused, the arteries leading into the penis open up so that pressurized blood can enter the penis quickly.
The veins leaving the penis constrict. Pressurized blood is trapped in the corpora cavernosa, and this blood causes the penis to elongate and stiffen. The penis is now erect. If the arteries leading to the penis do not open properly, it is difficult or impossible for a man to become erect. This problem is the leading cause of erectile dysfunction (ED). To solve an erection problem when the cause is poor blood flow, you need to open the arteries. There are

natural safe non- invasive methods to achieve this goal. I will discuss these methods later.

In addition to producing sperm, the testicles also produce male hormones, including testosterone. Testosterone has a sizable effect on sexual desire, and, in turn, sexual desire is often the first stage in sexual arousal and erection.

If the testicles are removed and testosterone production slows or stops, then sexual desire typically decreases, and erections may be fewer or nonexistent.

The prostate is a gland that surrounds the urethra in men and produces about 30% of the fluid that makes up what is called ejaculate or "cum." It is also a gland that is particularly prone to cancer, especially as men age.

It is important to get regular prostate examinations if you are 50 years or older. Treatments for prostate cancer, including surgical removal of the prostate, can cause erectile dysfunction (an inability to get an erection). This is not because the prostate is necessary to have an erection, but most likely because of the nerve or blood vessel damage caused by surgery or radiation treatments. Psychological trauma can also result from prostate removal. It can be said more often, take care of your prostate if you still have one.

What are some of the most common causes of ED or impotency in males?

As you might expect there are numerous medical conditions that can render a healthy sexual warrior inert.

Behind the scenes, a lot goes into achieving an erection. When you're turned on, nerves fire in your brain and travel down your spinal cord to your penis. There, muscles relax and blood flows into the blood vessels. If all goes well, a firm penis is now ready for sex.

Unfortunately, all does not always go well. Many diseases their treatment can lead to erectile dysfunction (ED).

Injuries, lifestyle choices, and other physical factors are known to play a significant role. ED can often be treated, and finding the right cause can lead to successful treatment.

Diabetes: This chronic disease can damage the nerves and blood vessels that aid in getting an erection. When the disease has not been well controlled over time, it can double a man's risk of erection problems.

Kidney Disease: Kidney disease can affect many of the things you need for a healthy erection, including your hormones, blood flow to your penis, and parts of your nervous system. It can also sap your energy level and rob you of your sex drive. Drugs for kidney disease can also cause ED.

Neurological Disorders: You can't get an erection without help from your nervous system. Diseases that disrupt signals between your brain and your penis can lead to ED. Such diseases include stroke, multiple sclerosis (MS), Alzheimer's disease, and Parkinson's disease.

Blood Vessel Diseases: Vascular diseases can block the blood vessels. That slows the flow of blood to the penis, making an erection difficult to get. Atherosclerosis (hardening of the arteries), high blood pressure, and high cholesterol are among the most common causes of ED.

Prostate Cancer: Prostate cancer doesn't cause ED, but treatments can lead to temporary or permanent erectile dysfunction.

The physical causes of ED are not only just disease-related. There are many other potential causes such as surgery. Surgery for both prostate cancer and bladder cancer can damage nerves and tissues necessary for an erection. Sometimes the problem may clear up within 6 to 18 months or the damage can be more permanent. If that happens, treatments are available to help restore a man's ability to have an erection.

Injury: Injuries to the pelvis, bladder, spinal cord, and penis that require surgery also can cause ED.

Hormone Problems: Testosterone and other hormones fuel a man's sex drive, and an imbalance can throw off his interest in sex.

Causes can include pituitary gland tumors, kidney and liver disease, depression, and hormone treatment of prostate cancer.

Venous Leak: To keep an erection, the blood that flows into your penis must stay in your penis. If it flows back out too quickly a condition called venous leak can occur. When the veins in your penis don't constrict properly you will lose your erection. Both injuries and disease can cause venous leak.

Tobacco, Alcohol, or Drugs: All three can damage your blood vessels. That makes it difficult for blood to reach the penis, which is essential for an erection. If you have hardened arteries (arteriosclerosis), smoking will dramatically raise your risk of ED.

Prescription Drugs: There are more than 200 prescription drugs that can cause ED as a result of their side effects.

Prostate Enlargement: Prostate enlargement, a normal part of aging for many men, may also play a role in ED.

We can clearly see that the enemy can come from within and without. The sexual warrior must be aware of the disabling or crippling power of these medical conditions and strive to avoid or prevent them. One must never give up hope to cure or mitigate these conditions. There are also emotional or psychological issues that can be just as devastating as the medical problems.

Erectile Dysfunction can also be caused by emotional problems:
Worry
Fear
Stress
Anger
Depression
Lack of interest in sex, or in the sexual partner

Good or Bad Testosterone

All forms of testosterone are not the same. A good comparison to testosterone is cholesterol. DHT or dihydrotestosterone is even more potent than testosterone itself in giving a man strong androgenic qualities like six pack, libido and lean muscle mass. Both forms of testosterone are good for a man. Now let'ss compare this to cholesterol.

 Most people are keenly aware that cholesterol can be good or bad. The bad cholesterol is called LDL. The good cholesterol is called HDL. Most doctors prefer patients have a higher ratio of HDL to LDL to help prevent heart disease. Cholesterol in itself is a very beneficial substance to the body. Most of our hormones are made from cholesterol.

The normal to healthy range is 130 -200 for total cholesterol profile.

What is considered to be the normal range is disputable. Many life and health insurance companies cholesterol reference scores for acceptability falls within the

200-300 range. A cholesterol of 245 may be optimal if the ratio of LDL to HDL is good. Higher HDL levels tend to neutralize the bad LDL.

Reference:

DiMeo PJ. Psychosocial and relationship issues in men with erectile dysfunction. Urol Nurs. 2006 Dec;26(6):442-6, 453; quiz 447.
Tikkanen MJ, Jackson G, Tammela T, et al. Erectile dysfunction as a risk factor for coronary heart disease: implications for prevention. Int J Clin Pract. 2007 Feb;61(2):265-8.
  Booth A, Johnson DR, Granger DA. Testosterone and men's health. J Behav Med. 1999; 22:1-19

Chapter 4

Sex Hormones and Enzymes

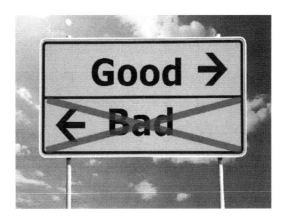

When we examine testosterone, we can easily find similar comparisons. Testosterone can come in several forms. The good and most beneficial. The most beneficial form of testosterone is called (DHT), which stands for dihydrotestosterone. This most potent and beneficial form of testosterone can sometimes be called free flowing or bio-available testosterone vs bounded testosterone(BT), unavailable to be used by the body.

Free flowing testosterone (FFT) comprises at best of only 2% of a man's total testosterone and is responsible for 95% of his sex drive, erectile strength and muscular lean body mass. When it comes to hormones 2% is a great deal. According to most medical lab results, the norms for the healthy total testosterone reference range is

250-1,000 ng/dl: for the free flowing, 35-155 pg/ml.

The good news about DHT is that it cannot be aromatized and converted into estrogen (estradiol). In the past DHT was considered a rogue version of testosterone that was often indicted into being associated with prostate enlargement.

Dihydrotestosterone (DHT)

Numerous new research studies indicate that DHT is even a more potent form of testosterone by comparison when it comes to enhancing male sexual potency. Below is a summary of this research:

- DHT is the most potent androgen in our body, 10-50 times more than testosterone itself.
- Can't be aromatized, and may even inhibit aromatization.
- DHT is the primary hormone for libido.
- Testosterone is converted into DHT via the enzyme 5-Alpha Reductase.
- DHT levels are often associated with androgenic male pattern baldness or alopecia, prostate enlargement. BPH is more the result of high estrogen level than DHT.
- Teenage boys should be the ones going bald, when these hormones are typically at their peak. This is not the case.

- Research shows that most men with male pattern baldness have low total testosterone, but with more of it free and more DHT available.

As you can see, DHT is now considered the welcomed friend rather than a foe. It has gotten a bad reputation by being blamed as the cause of male pattern baldness. My personal viewpoint on this issue is as follows:

- God only made a few real good men and the rest of them have hair.
- Younger women and men tend to over rate the presence of hair as a symbol of masculinity.
- The word bald originates from an old English word that means white. The bald eagle is not without hair on its head. Its head is just white.
- Many of the sexiest men in Hollywood are bald. Examples: The Rock, LL Cool Jay and
- Jason Statham and Patrick Stewart of Star Trek

Now we know that Dihydrotestosterone and Testosterone are both responsible of all masculine body and facial characteristics (wide jaw, broad shoulders...)
- *Increased DHT levels are strongly linked to higher brain GABA-levels, promoting that calm "alpha male" relaxation in any situation*
- *DHT (being the main androgen in male sexual organs) is even more potent than*

testosterone at promoting libido and erection quality

- If you are having prostate issues and are going bald, it's more likely that you possess the genotype for those conditions rather than high DHT.

Understanding Free vs Total Testosterone

Free and total testosterone should be carefully evaluated. Normal levels of testosterone for younger and older men reflect population averages. Most men would prefer not to accept the lost of sexual prowess as normal. A more valid reference range should be associated with men who are healthy and in the 21-49 age group. Looking at the chart below one can reference his levels in accordance to relative age. What is normal and healthy is relative. A man's ability to engage in a mutually satisfying sexual encounter should be the most important factor considered.

The normal or reference range is based on pure statistical methodology and simply defines where the middle 95% of the men fall with respect to their testosterone level. The bottom 2.5% are considered to be low and the top 2.5% are considered to be high.

If your testosterone level falls within the range of the middle 95% of the population you are considered to have "normal" testosterone levels. Normal levels only reflect the absence of disease. Optimal levels are those required for peak efficiency, function and prevention of age-related decline.

Contrary to what most believe, men like women also produce a form of estrogen called estradiol. The healthy reference range for men is 21.80-30.11 pg/ml. The human growth hormone also plays an important role in maintaining healthy testosterone levels and physical strength. The Hgh normal range should be 1,000-4,000 pg/ per 24 hour period.

All men should strive for optimal levels of testosterone rather than settling for what is considered normal.

Normal testosterone levels in men can vary from one lab to another. Adding to this confusion is the fact that there is more than one form of testosterone to be measured such as total testosterone and free testosterone. Testosterone in itself is almost useless in comparison to functional testosterone levels. Functional testosterone is referred to as called bio-available testosterone (BAT).

SHBG (sex hormone binding globulin) tends to rise with age and can render free testosterone useless if not kept under control. Later we will see why the supplementation and cycling is important for maintaining adequate levels throughout the day. One of the key supplements we will explore later in this book is known as Tongkat Ali.

There are herbal compounds in Tongkat Ali that limits the action of SHBG thus allowing for more (BAT) to be available when needed. Tongkat Ali is considered safe and natural.

Measurements in Conventional Units (ng/dl), SHBG in (nmol/L)

Age	# of Subjects	Total Test	Standard Dev.	Free Test	Standard Dev.	SHBG	Standard Dev.
25-34	45	617	170	12.3	2.8	35.5	8.8
35-44	22	668	212	10.3	1.2	40.1	7.9
45-54	23	606	213	9.1	2.2	44.6	8.2
55-64	43	562	195	8.3	2.1	45.5	8.8
65-74	47	524	197	6.9	2.3	48.7	14.2
75-84	48	471	169	6	2.3	51	22.7
85-100	21	376	134	5.4	2.3	65.9	22.8

<u>What are Sex Hormone Binding Globulin?</u>
Sex hormone–binding globulin (SHBG) modulates the bioavailability of sex steroids at tissue level. Genetic, hormonal and lifestyle-related factors determine the SHBG levels. Low SHBG levels are a known risk factor

for the development of the metabolic syndrome, diabetes and cardiovascular diseases.

The liver does all sorts of wonderful things in our lives; it metabolizes human growth hormone into IGF-1 and IGF-2, it filters toxins from the blood, it helps to regulate the flow of insulin from the pancreas to name a few. Part of its function is also to release a protein called sex hormone binding globulin (SHBG) in an effort to keep sex hormone levels like testosterone from becoming too high. Sometimes, the liver does its job too well, producing more SHBG than is needed. The result is that testosterone gets locked up and carried away before the body has a chance to use it. Testosterone exists in 2 states in the body: free and bound.

Free testosterone is the testosterone that our bodies use to build muscle, produce pheromones, maintains health and libido. It is the stuff that dreams are made of, the holy grail of the male sexual warrior.

Bound testosterone, on the other hand, has no bioavailability. It simply attaches itself to a protein, floating around the bloodstream. Bound testosterone does not interact well with any receptors in the body. Eventually, it becomes junk and is removed by the liver.

If your blood test showed up with low free testosterone, high bound testosterone, and low estrogen, then you are likely a victim of SHBG.

The condition is not likely to get better unless you are willing to be proactive. We cannot live very long without a liver due to its multitude of functions. It is best to leave this organ alone and treat the SHBG in the bloodstream instead.

Any alteration of liver function can have a domino effect on the rest of the body.

The most effective way of neutralizing SHBG comes not from the pharmacy, but from the roots of a common weed called Urtica Dioica, or more commonly called stinging nettle. It is interesting that a plant which is so hated by farmers and outdoorsmen offers an inexpensive and safe solution to such a terrible problem.

You could go on an herbal pilgrimage with a shovel, gloves and hiking boots to harvest roots and prepare your own extract. But if you are not up for the discomforts, you can easily pick some extract up at a health food store instead. There are several dietary supplements geared for men and men's health that include stinging nettle root and are very reasonably priced when weighed against the benefits that they provide.

What is DHEA?

DHEA, dehydroepiandrosterone, is an adrenal steroid hormone in the body. It is made by the adrenal glands and is then converted to androgens, estrogens and other hormones. These are the hormones that regulate fat and mineral metabolism, sexual and reproductive function, and energy levels. DHEA levels normally increase until our mid to late 20's then gradually start to decline.

DHEA, a precursor to testosterone, has been considered a significant nutrient to help support anabolic growth factors, increase muscle mass, reduced body fat and sexual enhancement. By the time your 65, your body only produces 10% of the DHEA that it produced when you were 20. That's why supplementation of DHEA is so vital for experiencing lower stress, staying healthier, and living longer.

DHEA production in the body may also decrease with the use of certain medications such as insulin and corticosteroids. DHEA is also thought to contribute to a sense of well-being when used by those with adrenal and or androgen insufficiency. In one placebo-controlled trial, DHEA supplementation for a 6-month period supported healthy physical and psychological outlook in men and women at ages 40-70 years. It may also support lean body mass in men and postmenopausal women. In another study, DHEA supplementation supported healthy male sexual function. The herb Tribulus is also a good source for improving one's DHEA levels.

Erectile Dysfunction – Taking DHEA orally for 24 weeks seems to improve ED, orgasmic function, sexual desire, and overall sexual satisfaction in men with erectile dysfunction secondary to hypertension. It may not be as beneficial in those with diabetes or neurological conditions.

Now let's look at what happens when things are not going well starting with the next question.

What are the 3 erection killer enzymes?

Men should be aware that there are enzymes lurking in the body waiting to receive a signal to kill their erection and sex life.

All sexual warriors should be able to identify and mount a strategy to control and suppress function of these enzymes. As men age, there are a number of biochemical processes that can become unbalanced. Let us begin with testosterone conversion. Healthy testosterone can be converted into estrogen by an enzyme called **aromatase**.

Aromatase converts testosterone into estrogen which can cause the prostate to become enlarged. This condition is often referred to as benign prostatic hypertrophy or BPH. A swollen prostate can cause a man to have frequent urination trips to the bathroom especially at night.

Although normally not a life death type of problem it can lead to cellular changes that can cause cancer of the prostate. During normal sexual activity, a man's prostate will usually undergo a series of contractions after an orgasm, thus returning it to normal size.

The aromatase enzyme interferes with this process. Male boobs called gynecomastia and fat accumulation can also be associated with the aromatase conversion of testosterone into DHT and estrogen. Men tend to become more estrogen dominant and effeminate in appearance. The good news is that aromatase can be controlled and minimized in terms of its impact upon the prostate.

- The prostate requires testosterone to remain in healthy disease-free state. Another culprit indicted in this unholy conversion of testosterone to DHT is another rouge enzyme called 5 Alpha Reductase or 5AR. The 5AR enzyme can also contribute to hair loss or alopecia if DHT is in excess but can also be controlled or minimized with proper diet and herbal supplementation. Long-term, abstinence, 3 months can reduce serum T.

Abstinence and Ejaculation Recovery

- Short-term abstinence from ejaculations can slightly increase testosterone. (7 days,145% spike)
- Having an ejaculation does not acutely affect testosterone levels.
- Ejaculating to the point of "sexual exhaustion" can make it harder for your body to utilize testosterone and recover.

- Masturbation doesn't seem to affect testosterone levels in any significant manner.
- Sex with a person can boost testosterone levels significantly.
- Older men who have more sex have higher T levels.

The Hijackers of Male Sexual Health

- **SHBG** Sex hormone binding globulin that limits Free Testosterone Availability.
- Aromatase Conversion of (T) to Estrogen
- PDE-5 (phosphodiesterase Type 5) deactivates cGMP
- Endocrine Disrupters- Xeno-estrogens
- Under Functioning Endothelium Cells that limit Nitric Oxide production in the Corpus Cavernosa and Spongiosum.
- Shrinking Leydig Cells (Hypogonadism) in the Testes causing a lost of mass thus limiting the production of (T) or aging.
- Excess Pornography and low dopamine levels

Given this understanding, most men can attest that they now know what they are fighting against. The enemy within becomes transparent. Nevertheless, surrendering to these enemies is not an option for the sexual warrior.

References :

1. Vermeulen, A. (1996). Declining Androgens with Age: An Overview. In Vermeulen, A. & Oddens, & B. J. (Eds.), Androgens and the Aging Male (pp. 3-14). New York: Parthenon Publishing. - See more at: http://www.mens-hormonal-health.com/normal-testosterone-levels-in-men.html#sthash.xZn6kuDL.dpuf

2. DiMeo PJ. Psychosocial and relationship issues in men with erectile dysfunction. Urol Nurs. 2006 Dec;26(6):442-6, 453; quiz 447.

3. Tikkanen MJ, Jackson G, Tammela T, et al. Erectile dysfunction as a risk factor for coronary heart disease: implications for prevention. Int

J Clin Pract. 2007 Feb;61(2):265-8.

4. Booth A, Johnson DR, Granger DA. Testosterone and men's health. J Behav Med. 1999;22:1-19

5. Booth A, Mazur AC, Dabbs JM, Jr. Endogenous testosterone and competition: the effect of "fasting". Steroids. 1993;58:348-50. ↥

6. Booth A, Shelley G, Mazur A, Tharp G, Kittok R. Testosterone, and winning and losing in human competition. Horm Behav. 1989;23:556-71.6. Eur J Appl Physiol, 2013 Jul, 113(7):1783-92,

7. "Effect of acute DHEA administration on free testosterone in middle-aged and young men following high-intensity interval training.

8. Life Sciences, May 4 1987, 40(18)1761-1768, "Diet-hormone interactions: Protein/carbohydrate ratio alters reciprocally the plasma levels of testosterone and cortisol and their respective binding globulins in man"

9. Lund, BC, Bever-Stille KA, Perry PJ, "Testosterone and andropause: the feasibility of testosterone replacement therapy in elderly men." Pharmacotherapy, 1999 Aug; 19(8): 951-6.

10. The T-Factor: King Of Hormones, Almark Publishing 2005 Pg 51

Chapter 5

Semen, The Seeds of Life

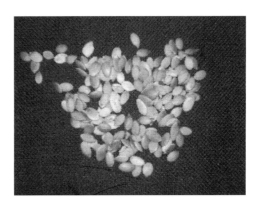

Semen derived from the Latin word seminis which means seed. It is truly the seed of life for men and should be treated with respect and guarded with care. How precious is a man's vital essence or semen? Many men assume that semen is an unlimited renewal resource like solar energy or wind and is virtually unlimited when it comes to sex. The problem lies more or less in quality and volume. After an ejaculation, there is a period of recovery needed to build up of sperm production. The period of recovery can range from 3-5 days for a healthy young fit male to a more extended time for an older maybe not so healthy male. Semen can be compared to oil as being necessary in the smooth functioning of a machine.

Semen is a man's oil, energy source and potential.

Semen contains sperm or the male seed of life. It is in a sense a man's vital essence that can be used for procreation, recreation and the re-creation of self. Semen is produced by the prostate and is the fluid that serves as a medium for sperm cells. The volume of semen can diminish or fluctuate depending upon a man's health, age or vitality. When men are young they are all but too willing to expend semen in a sexual encounter or orgasm. These men can be referred to as big spenders of vital essence.

As men age, many notice gradual changes in their health and sexual ability as they continue to expend large volumes of semen on a frequent basis. Sexual decline becomes almost inevitable which is linked to the ratio and frequency of semen loss. After many years of personal observations and interviews with various men, I am convinced that indiscriminate ejaculation is not good for men's health. As I mentioned earlier, once semen is released during a sexual orgasm there is a recovery period needed to replenish its loss.

During this interval, libido and vitality tend to decline depending upon a man's age. Energy levels are not as robust in comparison to having a full tank of gas prior to ejaculation. This is probably why most sport coaches forbid their athletes from having sex prior to or near the time of a competitive event. Most coaches fear that their athletes would suffer a lost of stamina, focus and drive for winning a competition.

How important is semen to a man's body?

According to Chinese medicine, one drop of semen is equal in vitality to 100 drops of blood. Another equivalent standard of measurement is based upon the ounce. An ounce of semen is considered to be equal in value to sixty ounces of blood and has the nutritional value of a large meal fit for an Olympic swimmer. Semen constitutes an extract of some of the most valuable of life sustaining compounds known to man.

The average male tends to ejaculate about one tablespoon of semen per orgasm. According to modern scientific research, the nutritional value of this amount is equal to two pieces of New York steak, ten eggs, six oranges and two lemons combined. It is indeed a nutrient dense elixir that profiles proteins, vitamins, mineral, sugars and hormones and more.

Semen also contains a great deal of vital energy or qi. An ejaculation can also represent a significant lost of vital energy. This is probably why men tend to feel so exhausted after sex while craving sleep in the aftermath.

The slang sexual term call" Cum or Coming" should be rephrased as" Going or Gone" with regards to the amount

of energy expended. A man can lose virtually everything from erection, vital energy, sperms, hormones, nutrients and desire in one grand ejaculatory explosion. In reality the very act of ejaculation becomes a great sacrifice for a man spiritually, mentally and physically when done in excess.

Moderation of ejaculation is good first step for most men in an attempt to preserve their vital essence. The best most enduring solution is injaculation of semen into the body for the recycling of the life force and male potency.

The ancient Chinese Taoist and Hindu Sexual Tantra Masters have long practiced these methods for many years thus achieving higher consciousness and supreme wellness of mind, body and spirit. Based upon Mantak Chia's book the Taoist Secret of Love, 1986 edition, he clearly stresses how precious sperm or sexual energy is for maintaining our health and sexual readiness. He states that 25% to 40% of our chi or qi energy is received from food, water, air and sunlight to generate sexual energy. Production of this nutrient rich fluid requires a great deal of raw material. It is the blood that extracts this material from every part of the body, kidneys, liver, endocrine glands and even the brain.

According to the Kinsley Report, the average male ejaculates 5,000 times in his lifetime. This would be the equivalence of 4 gallons. No man should take his semen for granted and expend it without thought of health consequences.

Like most men, I too became interested in knowing the biochemical nutrient content of semen. This is the reason I decided to use the picture of pumpkin seeds as an opener for this chapter due to its high content of zinc. The nutrient zinc is vital for the production of healthy sperm cells in men of all ages. Men should strive to understand how important the nutrient composition of semen is when viewed from the perspective of vitamins/minerals. This valuable information is now available to all. The following data was collected from my research on the 1992 World Health Organization nutrient profile of semen. Ok, brace yourself to the following.

The composition of semen is as follows:
Testes: 2-5%. Approximately 200- to 500-million spermatozoa (also called sperm or spermatozoans are present in the testes and are released per ejaculation. Seminal vesicle: 65-75% amino acids, citrate, enzymes, flavins, fructose (the main energy source of sperm cells, which rely entirely on sugars from the seminal plasma for

energy), phosphorylcholine and prostaglandins (involved in suppressing an immune response by the female against

foreign semen.)

Prostate: 25-30% acid phosphatase, citric acid, fibrinolysin, prostate specific antigen, proteolytic enzymes, zinc (serves to help to stabilize the DNA-containing chromatin in the sperm cells. A zinc deficiency may result in lowered fertility because of increased sperm fragility. Zinc deficiency can also adversely affect spermatogenesis.

Bulbourethral glands < 1% galactose, mucus serve to increase the mobility of sperm cells in the vagina and cervix by creating a less viscous channel for the sperm cells to swim through. These glands prevent the diffusion of sperms out of the semen. This mucus contributes to the cohesive jelly-like texture of semen.

World Health Organization report describes normal human semen as having a volume of 2 ml or greater, pH of 7.2 to 8.0, sperm concentration of $20x10^6$ spermatozoa/ml or more, sperm count of $40x10^6$ spermatozoa per ejaculate or more and motility of 50% or more with forward progression. This degree of motility all occurs within a 60 minutes window of ejaculation. On the following is a break down of the nutrient composition of semen.

The Nutrient Composition of Semen
Seminal fluid... is composed of dozens of chemical components. The
base of seminal fluid is primarily fructose (sugar) and proteins, with
many other trace minerals and substances.
Here's a listing of some of
ingredients in semen:

Sugars: Fructose, sorbitol, inositol
Proteins and amino acids: glutathione, deoxyribonucleic acid (DNA), creatine
Minerals: Phosphorus, zinc, magnesium, calcium, potassium
Vitamins: Ascorbic acid (vitamin C), vitamin B12, choline
Hormones: Testosterone, prostaglandins
Body byproducts: Lactic acid, urea, uric acid, nitrogen...
Semen is a source of highly concentrated, high-quality protein. In
dietary terms, it's comparable to egg whites or gelatin. Besides
protein, semen contains high concentrations of some minerals, such as zinc, and trace amounts of other important nutrients, like calcium and
magnesium.

Now that we know how nutrient dense and precious the vital fluid of life is, it is important to monitor indiscriminate loss without sacrificing pleasure. The solution to this problem has already been explored and documented by the masters of India and China. This topic will be discussed in the next chapter.

References:

Dr. Stephan Chang, The Tao of Sexology, Tao publishing
1. 1986, pg. 63

2. Mantak Chia, Taoist Secrets of Love, Aurora Press, 1984.

Wikipedia definition of semen/ Review of the Physical and Chemical Properties of Human Semen and the Formulation of a Semen Simulant

Derek H. Owen[*] and David F. Katz
Article first published online:
JAN 2013DOI: 10.2164/jandrol.04104

Chapter 6

Conservation of Semen and Testicle Massage

In ancient India and Chin, the practice of preserving the vital essence of the body was called Tantra Yoga. In China, it is simply referred to as The Seminal Retention Method or Sexual Kung-fu. According to Daniel Reid, Author of "The Tao of Health Sex & Longevity" semen essence is the fuel that drives male sexuality. It is the source not only of physical capacity for sex, but also of sexual interest and emotional affection for the opposite gender.

Both methods employ the same principles of conserving the vital seed and transmuting it into energy qi, longevity and enhanced awareness. Let us now explore some options for conservation of semen that have been practiced in the past.

The first aspect of semen retention for men starts with simply learning to control involuntary ejaculation. By using authentic tantra retention methods men can learn to manage their sexual responses, and prolong sexual stimulation if they choose. These unique methods can contribute to the mental and emotional health of a man by giving him a sense of personal empowerment with regards to his sexuality. He will in time develop a deeper sense of self-confidence in being able to sexually satisfy his partner.

Another important benefit of semen retention may very well be an increased sex drive. A recent study from China shows that seminal retention can increase testosterone levels by 45.7% after 7 days. According to this method, a man who maintains consistently high levels of testosterone by practicing ejaculatory control will experience an overwhelming enhancement in the love and affection for his woman. He will also gain the capacity to act upon that loving urge repeatedly.

In Tibetan medicine, it is said that "seven drops of the vital essence of food are required to produce one drop of the vital essence of blood. It takes one cup of the vital essence of blood to produce one drop of the vital essence of semen.

Taoist Sexual Master Mantak Chia has stated that when men retain their semen during sexual activity, their brain energy increases double fold. He also states that semen contains substances of high physiological value, especially in relation to the nutrition of the brain and nervous system.

 Their may be some truth after all to the common phrase of "fucking your brain out" due to excessive indiscriminate ejaculation. A natural health consultant, Jacque Drouin and Founder of Authentic Tantra, recommends an ejaculation frequency of once every 6 weeks for his male students, over the age of 35. He says that "initially it takes a good 6 weeks for the body to begin to regenerate after a lifetime of chronic, unregulated ejaculation and for male power to really begin to build."

I find it interesting that men and women are only able to donate blood once every 6 weeks, yet it is considered normal and "healthy" in western medicine & sexology for a man to ejaculate as often as every day. I am sure that there is a strong correlation in terms of the 6- week seminal make-over period.

Correct application of semen retention method can help men achieve multiple consecutive orgasms. It is important to that understand that orgasm and ejaculation are two separate functions of the nervous system. Many men tend to confuse the two and misjudge the effectiveness of this method.

After years of exhaustive research on the hot topic of conservation of semen, I discovered that there exist various methods and approaches that can be distilled into 4 fundamental approaches. The first to be discussed is what I call the "Breast Milk Semen Connection." Lets us now draw a comparison of the two. Breast and testicles/prostate are remarkably similar in function and design. Both organs are secreting glands and part of the endocrine glandular system. A woman's breast milk is produced by mammary glands in response to the necessity of feeding her baby. Both semen and beast milk are nutrient dense with similar composition. If a woman decides to breast feed, her body will produce a quantity of milk that is in proportion to the need of her baby. In other words, the more the baby sucks the more breast milk is stimulated and produced. This process is highly influenced by the hormone, prolactin.

On the other hand, if a woman chooses to stop breast feeding her milk supply will gradually diminish. Let us compare this event to semen. Both breast milk and semen are produced by secreting glands that can become engorged when stimulated. The more the testicles are stimulated the more sperms are produced as well as the seminal fluid. It is a medical fact that a man's testicle can shrink during prolonged periods of celibacy. In contrast, a woman's breast size as well as her supply of milk decreases when she abstains from breast feeding. A simple way of viewing this action can be summed up as the use it or lose it principle.

In conclusion, it appears that supply and demand dictates heavily and influences the production of both semen and breast milk. It would also seem that the more the body places demand upon itself, the more the body produces to keep up with demand. I am sure there is a point of diminishing returns if this approach is taken to extremes.

The second practice, although somewhat esoteric is called the <u>Taoist Seminal Retention Method</u> (TSR). Today in modern terms, we call this method, Edging. The TSR method recommends that a man should retain his semen and not ejaculate during a sexual intercourse in exchange for greater vitality, increased testosterone, stronger future erections and sexual stamina.

This approach is somewhat esoteric for the average man and can have some draw backs if not mastered within a reasonable amount of time. One drawback is the swelling of the prostate that occurs during sex along with the engorgement of semen. Over time the lack of flushing of the prostate could lead to unhealthy cellular changes possibly cancer as well as a swollen prostate that lacks proper muscle tone. When the prostate stays enlarged over an extended period it can lead to a condition called benign prostatic hypertrophy (BPH) triggering the need for frequent urinations for men especially at night. Edging can however still be practiced safely in moderation.

What is Edging or Orgasm Without Ejaculation?

Edging is the art of having micro orgasms.

It is a technique that requires a man to restrain himself just prior to ejaculation or full orgasm

Each time the temptation to ejaculate is controlled the testicles become more able to produce a little more sperm and testosterone.

Over time a heighten surge of sexual energy begins to build up inside you.

What you do with this energy is entirely up to you.

Most men will orgasm, every single time, at the end of an edging session.

We save up the orgasms, the sperm, the testosterone, and the sexual energy to be able to function at a more intense level when the situation dictates.

Edging is a powerful technique that a sexual warrior should have in his arsenal.

The Taoist states that a special spot or the male G Spot have to be pressed or manipulated by means of muscle control or thought. The G Spot is the control valve for semen to be injaculated back into the body instead of ejaculated and wasted. This spot is sometimes referred to as the "Million Dollar Point" by Dr. Stephen Chang, in his book on The Tao of Sexuality. He states that The Male G Spot or The Huiyin Point according to Chinese Acupuncture Medicine is the master switch of ejaculation control. This special point can be located by feeling for a spot half way between the anus and the testicles that is slightly sunken. It takes much practice and patience to master this method and sometimes can interfere with the flow of things.

The third method is called <u>The Age and Frequency Method</u>. According to this method, a man should only ejaculate in an interval that is appropriate for his age. By doing so, he can maintain his health, longevity and sexual prowess well into advanced age. It is said that this method can also slow or retard the aging process of his body. There is a mathematical formula that Dr. Stephen Chang, The Tao of Sexology, highlights in his book. The formula stated that the optimal schedule for ejaculation should be based upon a man's age x .2. For example, if a man is 20 years of age, multiply 20 x .2= 4.0 days. This is the average amount of time needed for replenishing his semen. On or after the fourth day since his previous ejaculation he is permitted to release semen without any negative health consequences. In contrast, if a man is 60 years of age he should wait at least 12 days after his previous release of semen   before releasing again, 60 x .2=12.0 days.

The fourth and final approach is a combination of the previous methods stated which entail scheduled release and Edging. I personally prefer scheduled ejaculation combined with the use of Edging in moderation. Done properly both methods can impart health benefits while avoiding the negative medical side effects of the seminal retention method practiced in extreme. I believe that moderation is the key to longevity and health in contrast to indiscriminate use of extreme measures which are often without virtue. The rules for scheduled release are flexible and can be adjusted according to the overall health and vitality of a man. Instead of a healthy 60 year old man waiting 12 days he may only need to abstain for 10 days.

Why is Testicle Massaging Important?

Testicle Massage improves the blood circulation to the testicles, which can also boost production of testosterone during the recovery period between sexual encounters.

According to Mantak Chia's book, Taoist Secrets of Love, massaging your testicles regularly will improve erection, ejaculation and volume of sperm. Testicle massage will even increase the size of your testicles thus making them fuller more dense and sensitive.

Testicles are very vital and important organs in a man's body and without them we would become an extinct

species. Keeping them in top notch shape will not only give you harder erections, more sex drive, and higher volume of ejaculation. Healthy robust testicles are necessary to have for a healthier sperm count and a better chance to procreate to children.

Does Testicle Massage Increase Testosterone Levels?

Healthy, normal testicles produce somewhere between 4-7 mg of testosterone a day. Since you're reading this now, chances are you may only be producing about 1-2 mg a day.

Adding massage to your routine will help you improve those numbers. Benefits of Testicle Massage are as follows:

Elevated Testosterone Levels

Enhanced Erections

Increased Ejaculation Volume

Enhanced Circulation to the Testes

Elevated Sperm Count

The key to proper testicle function and health is better blood circulation to your testicles.

The following exercises below explain how to increase a higher-level blood circulation to your testicles to promote all round better function and health. Remember, testicle massaging should never be painful. Before doing anything, apply a nice warm moist wrap to your testicles for about 5 minutes.

This will make them warm and the skin more pliable to stretch and massage. After using the warm wrap apply a healthy dousing of olive oil into your palms and really work it into your testicles skin, covering all viable areas with olive oil. Make sure the oil is really rubbed into the skin.

Begin to massage all surrounding areas of your testicles, but not the testicles directly. Massage in between your testicles with a pumping motion using your thumb and fingers.

Massage at the base, pulling down as you massage.

Do this for about 3 minutes. Take your hands with your fingers spread apart and grip your testicles at the root and lightly pull them down, bring them back up, them pull them down again, over and over for about 3 minutes.

Lightly apply pressure to your testicles, massaging them while doing so. Massage all around them, working your way around both of your testicles. Continue to repeat all of these steps over and over again.

This massaging routine should be done for at least 10 minutes a day, preferably in the morning or before bedtime. A minimum massage of 3 times a week should stretch out your testicle skin real well while feeling a good stretch as you pull the skin down. Another good stretching method similar to The Testicle Power Stretch is the Grasping Method.

Grasp around the base of your testicles with your thumb and forefinger and squeeze until your testicles are tight together on top of your thumb and forefinger. Take the other hand and apply a small amount of pressure on top of the testicles and massage them in a circular motion. While you are doing this, pull down lightly the hand that is grabbing the base of your testicles connecting flesh.

Do this for about 3-5 minutes without stopping.
After these massaging exercises, your testicles should be stretched out and appear to be hanging lower than normal, as well as appearing to be larger. This is due to the increased blood circulated into your testicles from performing the above exercises. You should do these massaging and stretching techniques at least 3-4 times a week, but daily exercise can be performed for absolute optimal testicle health and fertility.

In summary, I believe that each method is valid and needs to be tailored to the individual according to his needs, constitutional type and lifestyle. It is also important for a man to be able to increase his production of sperm and volume of semen to satisfy any demand. When it comes to improving sexual health the message is clear. A man must be proactive. While conservation may be important, making a surplus of sperms and semen can keep a man on top of his game without fear of diminished vitality. It is in my opinion, that it is better to be in a position to have more than you need and spend.

I called this approach,

"The Pump Up The Volume Method." Increasing volume of sperm is equally as important as conserving semen by utilizing some of the previous methods mentioned. Supplementation with vital tonic herbs such as Polyrachis, He Shou Wu, and Cordyceps can have a very positive effect on increasing the volume

and quality of sperm/semen production. Internal breathing meditative exercises such as yoga, qi gong, tai chi chuan should also be considered. The best approach, in my opinion, combines the judicious use of herbs with internal exercises to create a more powerful synergistic effect.

References :

Dr.Stephan Chang, The Tao of Sexology,Tao publishing 1986, pg. 63

Mantak Chia, Taoist Secrets of Love, Aurora Press,1984

Chapter 7

The Seasonal Cycles of Sex

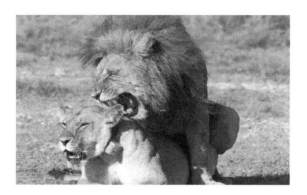

Nature often reveals many secrets to us if we are only observant enough. The ancient sages tend to view mankind as a microcosm of the macrocosmic universe. They learned from thousand of years of empirical studies that the outer processes of nature quite often mimic those that occur in man. One of the processes worth highlighting is the law of cycles. The law of cycles shows no favoritism to any one life form apart from another. Knowing that these laws exist help us know what to expect.

The law of cycles states that events happen in a repetitive pattern of increase, stability, decrease and then increase again. Our ancestors knew about the law of cycles much better than we do today. They were keenly aware that during certain periods food was more plentiful and in others scarce. They were aware of changes in weather patterns such as severe storm patterns. Dramatic population cycles for certain animals would fluctuate from high to low depending upon available resources.

Despite challenging conditions, nature's clock always seems to find a way of balancing itself by restoring the polar side of the cycle when change is eminent.

Nowadays, we tend to lose sight of this basic law of nature. In this century, we have grown to rely on our national government and technology to solve most of our problems. The stock market on Wall Street is also subjected to the law of cycles. We generally believe that our standard of living, income, health and well-being should always improve as a function of technology.

Cycles are an inevitable part of life. We must learn how to use it to our advantage. According to the law of cycles even bad conditions will eventually improve, so patience is better than complaint. The idea of cycles shows the importance of timing. Now you might be asking the questions how do cycles relates to sexual readiness? There are two major components to answering this question.

Good quality sex is based upon one's biorhythms and timing. Let us first investigate the impact of timing. When is the best season to have sex?

The answer should not surprise you. The best times for men to have sex are during the spring and summer seasons. Spring in itself, is a natural aphrodisiac.

During these seasons, the sap rises in trees. Flowers begin to bloom and many animals awaken from hibernation to mate. Internally, our bodies also experience the four seasons just as nature does because

we are all are part of nature.

The rising of the sap in the trees can be equated to our hormonal fluids surging during this time signaling our brains to produce more sperm cells. The next big question is not so friendly. When is the worst time to have sex for men? The answer is during the winter season. Men should not expect or place high demands on their bodies to perform like a stud horse during this time. For many men, a dip or decline in sexual performance does not necessarily signal a problem. The best explanation for this decline is merely a seasonal shift of sexual energy into hibernation mode for rejuvenation and rest.

According to Chinese medicine, the winter cycles in itself, embodies what is referred to as the 4 Depleting Yin Qi Energies. They are coldness, dampness, wind and darkness or a shorter day cycle.

Sex by its nature is considered to be yang and warming thus requiring much inner heat and vitality. During the winter period, surplus yang energy is usually deficient because our bodies must compensate for the loss of heat in an effort to maintain core body temperature.

We also need to build outer resistance to the penetrating effects of the four negative yin energies. The yin external conditions can easily undermine one's health, thus setting the stage for upper respiratory infections, flu, poor circulation and low libido.

The warrior's diet, sleeping habits, herbal supplements, and physical training must be adapted to the demands of the winter. Based upon the principles of the Chinese Five Element Theory, nature is in her resting cycle, quietly withdrawn deep into the earth. December 21 is the day of the winter solstice and the longest night during this cycle. Since days are shorter our bodies become more yin (subdued) at an earlier time. This would suggest that a man should have intercourse earlier during the day in the winter rather than waiting until evening. Early evening is also a better choice than late evening during the winter period.

Both nature and mankind are dominated by the Yin Principle. The organs most sensitive during the winter months are the kidneys and bladder.

The kidneys control the life force and sexual energy. Weak kidney energy may be experienced as lethargy, low vitality, weak knees and erectile dysfunction. Other manifestations can also include frequent urination, anxiety and low back pain. The kidneys and sex organs are ruled by the Yin Water Principle. A man should avoid having sexual relations during the winter at night when the weather conditions are extremely yin or inclement.

Men should not set their expectations or performance levels too high during this time. The winter season is the

best time to be more conservative. There are exceptions for those who live in a region where the climate is cold most of the time like Sweden. Given sufficient time a man's body will gradually adapt to cold weather. Internally, he will be able to generate more warmth and qi to offset the debilitating effects of winter. Men need to live close to nature by being outside often and avoid the overuse of technology to stay warm.

A good supplemental herb to take during the winter months or cold periods is cinnamon. Cinnamon can really warm things up when needed. This herb is sweet, spicy and warming in nature.

I recommend taking 1 teaspoon of powdered cinnamon in a cup of hot water at least 30 minutes prior to intercourse or at least twice daily. Ginger can also be taken as well. I personally prefer the use of cinnamon and have noticed good results from its usage. One exception to the yin rule is having intercourse at night during the full moon cycle.

The full moon is of a yang element present during the yin cycle of winter. The full moon lunar cycle tends to provide balance for the greater yin influence of the night. Men are on a solar cycle and women are on a lunar cycle. Getting an earlier evening start seems to work better when it comes to having sex during the winter. Another important measure for a man to take to preserve the sexual energy during the winter months would be to retire early and sleep in late. This simple practice alone can help to easily replenish the body's yang or vital surplus energy taxed by the winter months.

Much of our chi supply can easily be consumed during the winter just trying to stay warm leaving little in reserve for sex. As I stated earlier, don't push yourself physically hoping for more gain during the winter months.

Be conservative and save your best performance for spring. In this case, the paradox to be learned is less is more. Remember winter is a time to cultivate energy, qi and protect your vital reserves energy.

You are not a sex machine so don't try to be one. Be conservative and save your best performance for spring.

If a man wants to perform well sexually he must know his biorhythms or bio-cycles.

What are biorhythms? The history of biorhythms extends back to 3000 years ago. Scientists of ancient Greece began recording the regular rhythms of basic bodily functions such as respiration, kidney activity, pulse rate and, of course, libido. You can easily find examples of biorhythm charts online at:

www.biorhythmonline.com/comp.php

If you would like to calculate your own biorhythms and determine the best time for sex and times you should avoid it visit the following website

(http://www.biorhythm-calculator.net

Biorhythms are inherent cycles that affect you physically, emotionally and intellectually. They regulate metabolism, coordination, emotions, memory, sexuality, creativity and more.

As each of your biorhythm cycles rise and fall, so does your ability to perform certain tasks, physical activities, deal with stress, and make sound decisions.

Biorhythms are easy to understand, but hard to generalize. Everyone has gone from having a great day to having a bad day, yet this is not a collective experience but rather a personal one.

If you track your mood swings and your physical and intellectual highs and lows, then compare them to your biorhythms, you will begin to understand more about what makes you tick.

The Three Primary Biorhythm Cycles

Here is a detailed list of the three primary cycles and their respective durations. They are usually color coded to match international biorhythm standards:

Physical Biorhythm Cycle ~~ Red ~~ 23 days

The physical cycle is considered to be the dominant cycle for men. It regulates hand-eye coordination, strength, endurance, sex drive, initiative, metabolic rate, resistance to and recovery from illness. Surgery should be avoided on physical transition days and during negative physical cycles.

Emotional Biorhythm Cycle ~~ Blue ~~ 28 days

The emotional cycle is said to be the dominant cycle in women. It regulates emotions, feelings, mood, sensitivity, sensation, sexuality, fantasy, temperament, nerves, reactions, affections and creativity. Men should try being intimate with women during there optimal emotional cycle.

Intellectual Biorhythm Cycle ~~ Green ~~ 33 days
The intellectual cycle regulates intelligence, logic, mental reaction, alertness, sense of direction, decision-making, judgment, power of deduction, memory, and ambition.

Transition Days
Transition days are the day when a biorhythm cycle changes polarity.

At mid point and end point in each biorhythm cycle, the cycle sharply moves back to zero point and changes polarity. That is called a transition day (or caution, or critical day). As the cycles constantly change polarity, we experience life's ups and downs.

A double transition day is when 2 of your cycles change polarity on the same day. This day may be difficult, especially if both cycles are changing polarity in tandem (going in the same direction).

A triple transition day is when 3 of your cycles change polarity on the same day. Triple transition days are rare, occurring once every 7-8 years.

The toughest days are multiple transition days closely following each other. For example, JFK Jr left on his last flight during one of these phases. All 3 of his cycles had transitions within a 72-hour period, which would explain his high confidence level, yet lack of good judgment.

Each one of us has this combination several times a year. Sometimes this can happen once or twice in a one month period. Those days can really be challenging.

Positive and Negative Cycles (High and Low)

It is important that we do not turn negative transition days, and negative cycles, into a self-fulfilling prophecy. Negative cycles and transition days are necessary. For instance, when your intellectual cycle is low, your intuition may be at its peak. During a triple low cycle (all three cycles negative) your subconscious has more room to maneuver.

A triple low cycle is one of the best times to get in touch with your inner spirit and an excellent time to learn from insightful dreaming. Not a good time to go mountain climbing but rather time to take it easy and regenerate.

You may think having all three cycles in the positive would be great, but that's not true either. People who are experiencing a triple high can be pushy, irritating, and downright obnoxious (assuming that's not their usual temperament).

Confidence levels can be so high that disastrous mistakes may be made. Balance is the key!

Understanding your positive biorhythm cycles will assist you in planning sporting events, public activities, intellectual endeavors, even romance!
Understanding your negative biorhythm cycles can help you avoid accidents, hurtful situations, grief and misfortune.

Self Exploration

Biorhythm calendars can be an excellent tool for athletes, pilots, surgeons, lovers, actors, teachers, parents, and anyone wanting to know when their "off" days are approaching.

If you are interested in finding out more go to (http://biorhythmcalendar.com/wordpress/)

References:

The 5 Element Theory Chinese Medicine for Beginners: Use the Power of the Five Elements to Heal Body and Soul Paperback – October 2, 1996 by Achim Eckert

www.biorhythmonline.com/comp.php

www.biorhythmcalendar.com/wordpress

www.biorhythm-calculator.net

Chapter 8

THE LOW (T) MYTH AND PANIC

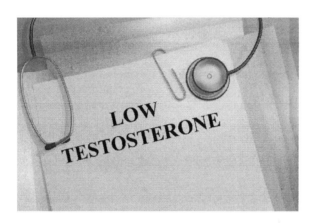

Low T refers to a man's inability to generate normal healthy levels of the hormone testosterone. It is sometimes referred to as testosterone deficiency syndrome or male andropause. Ultimately, it is the brain that determines how much testosterone is produced. A message from the hypothalamus to the pituitary gland sets the stage for action by the testes, the actual producers of testosterone. The adrenal glands also produce a small amount of testosterone thus contributing to what is known as the total testosterone.

Testosterone is the anabolic hormone that is formed in testes. It has a major impact on men's health, maintenance, growth of the male sex traits, increase in the level of protein anabolism and more.

Your bloodstream contains two types of testosterone: bonded testosterone and free testosterone sometimes called bioactive testosterone. Bonded testosterone attaches to molecules in the body and is mostly ineffective. However, the 'free' testosterone can enter your cells easily and play a vital role in libido strength, stamina, and vitality. In short, free testosterone helps a man be a man!

High free testosterone levels are linked to increased sex drive, a higher libido, and heightened desire. Maintaining an optimal free testosterone level is vital for men. High free testosterone levels can help with:
- Maximizing your gains in the gym
- Boosting libido and increasing desire
- Revitalizing drive and performance

Testosterone levels can vary throughout the day. A blood test is normally used to diagnose low testosterone. The testing is usually done in the early morning when the level peaks. A normal level is anything between 300 and 1200 ng/dl. A more ideal level range would be between 600-800.

When a man's testosterone level is too low, he may experience any of the following symptoms:

Decreased sex drive

Low sperm count

No, or inadequate, erections

Increased breast size
Hot flashes
Depression
Irritability
Difficulty concentrating

Similar symptoms can be seen in many other forms of illnesses including old fashion chronic stress.

When men opt to change their lifestyle for the better, many of these symptoms seem to diminish or cease to

cause problems. There's no single cause of testosterone deficiency. Aging can be a factor but is not the sole determinant. Testosterone levels can decrease about one percent per year after the mid-30s. Disease, accidental testicular cell damage, inflammation, and side effects of medical treatments may also lead to low testosterone levels. If these problems don't apply to you then avoid the unnecessary use of testosterone gels.

Low T gel can create a hormonal imbalance in a normal male with low testosterone creating a negative feedback loop. Once an external topical gel is used repeatedly over time a man's body will eventually begin to signal the pituitary gland and hypothalamus to decrease normal production. This is what I refer to as a medically induce low testosterone syndrome or more commonly a negative feedback loop.

In other words, the more you use the less your body produce naturally. Long term use of exogenous (non-natural) testosterone can dampen the body's natural production of testosterone, and men may require

treatment with **human chorionic gonadotropin, or HCG** (a natural precursor to testosterone) so that they can begin making testosterone naturally again.
Read: http://www.ehow.com/about_5383047_dangers-testosterone.html#ixzz2uvSfS8XI

Eventually, this process will cause a man to become totally dependent on synthetic testosterone gel. The use of Low T gel is definitely not a panacea to opt for early in the game. Men should strive to do a better job at understanding and exploring healthier options.
From a historical perspective, societal testosterone levels have dropped in the past 20 years. This may be explained in part by the side effects of medication and the rising obesity levels due to body fat conversion of testosterone into estrogen. Environmental toxins that mimic estrogens such as pesticides may also be partly to blame.

As mentioned earlier, stress can be a major cause of Low T. Chronic stress can shut down a man's libido and trigger the release of a hormone called cortisol. The cortisol produced in response to stress also interferes with one's insulin production. When cortisol levels increase, insulin resistance goes up and insulin sensitivity decreases. Increased cortisol levels are also associated with increase weight leading to obesity.

Once a man's production of fat cells increases, a similar increase in estrogen receptor sites are also noted as well.
 When the ratio of estrogen to testosterone is out of balance, a higher conversion of testosterone to estrogen tends to also occur.
 This process creates another negative vicious cycle of reduced free testosterone.
 Levels below 150 ng/dl are usually indicative of hypogonadism or Low T.

 The use of testosterone prescriptions has tripled since 2001 with men in their 40s representing the fastest-growing group of users. Only about half of men taking testosterone have an actual diagnosis of hypogonadism.
Even more curious, recent findings indicate that 25 percent of men given a prescription for testosterone did not even have their levels tested prior to receiving a prescription, and of the remaining 75 percent, it was unclear as to how many

had a testosterone deficiency.

In short, there appears to be an awful lot of men out there taking testosterone who probably shouldn't. Using hormones as a "cure-all" is a risky proposition, especially if your problems are related to lifestyle.

Keep in mind that there are actual medical conditions that can severely impair your hormone production. What most men need is really a lifestyle change to optimize their body's natural secretion of testosterone and other hormones.

According to one recent study published in the Journal PLOS One, men aged 65 and older who took testosterone doubled their risk of having a heart attack within the first three months of use. The majority of them did not have heart disease prior to starting the therapy. The result was similar in younger men diagnosed with heart disease. The study was prompted by a 2010 clinical trial that was shut down before completion due to the increase in heart-related problems occurring in the testosterone treatment group. While a man's testosterone level does decline with age, starting around the age of 30 there are many other factors that play a role. In past generations, men were more active and healthy well into old age.

It is possible to grow old without losing your mojo. Lifestyle, diet and exercise are also critical factors. But chemical exposures, including prescription drugs like statin, can also play a role by having an adverse effect on testosterone production in terms of side effects.

Testosterone appears to decline naturally with aging but internal belly fat depresses the hormone further, especially in obese men. Drugs like steroids and opiates can also lower testosterone.

It is suspected that chemicals like bisphenol A (or BPA, commonly found in plastic food containers) and diseases like Type 2 diabetes play a role as well.

These chemicals are responsible for the creation of what is called xenoestrogens. This type of estrogen represents one of the most destructive forms of synthetic hormonal compounds known to man. I call them the testosterone or "T Killers."

Testosterone production along with HGH, human growth hormone also tends to decline with age. Fortunately, our body does have a natural ability to optimize hormones, even as you age. In order to be successful, men need to address important key factors such as diet, attitude and exercise. A comprehensive plan of action tailored to one's true needs in addition to an all out committed effort can produce remarkable results. Both testosterone and HGH in men can rapidly decline after the age of 40 years.

For instance, in a 55-year-old male the rate of reduction of HGH can drop from 900 units to 400 units

as compared to a 30-year-old male in good health.

Research by many modern physiologists supports the conclusion that high intensity interval training is the best form of exercises for increasing both testosterone and HGH levels. A slow one-hour jog will not have this effect. Therefore, make sure you are exercising correctly if you want to make real gains and see visible results in a shorter period of time.

A 60 years old male's level of HGH is usually just 1/5th of what is produced by a 20 years old man. As per some experiments, introducing HGH in older men have resulted in a noticeable increase in the sexual desire, lean muscle mass as well as energy. An amazing level of improvements in testosterone were noticed as well.

How to do High Intensity Exercises

The best way to do (HIIT) or high intensity interval training is as follows:

Warm up for three minutes

Exercise as hard and fast as you can for 30 seconds. You should feel like you couldn't possibly go on another few seconds. Recover at a slow to moderate pace for 90 seconds. Repeat the high intensity exercise and recovery seven more times.

Weight training will also have a beneficial impact on both HGH and testosterone levels when done correctly. When you use strength training for this purpose, you'll want to increase the weight and lower your number of reps. Focus on doing exercises that work a wider number of muscles such as squats or dead lifts.

You can take your workout to the next level by learning the principles of super slow weight training or by incorporating the use of whole body vibration training using a power plate.

Many men naturally assume that their sexual decline issues are attributed to having symptoms of low T when in fact it may be due to low HGH. Low HGH can render a man impotent and saturated with a higher estrogen than testosterone level. Low HGH can lead to obesity and higher insulin levels and ultimately to clinical low T. Exactly how does HGH increase testosterone levels in men? Well the answer is just a little complicated. Well here it goes.

Natural HGH encourages your pituitary gland to generate more of the particular pure HGH. As soon as it is discharged directly into the system, the natural HGH starts revitalizing various systems of the body.

The main area of focus, the testicles, increase the generation of testosterone in order to improve muscle production and wake up your sexual desire. When HGH is replenished, testosterone levels are also impacted. This process is referred to as hormonal stacking.

The HGH testosterone stack has a compound effect, far greater than either of the two hormones individually. For example, testosterone helps the human growth hormone – HGH – work faster,
While increasing cellular efficiency and aiding recovery. The HGH testosterone stack also restores focus, energy, sex drive and performance to those levels of our youth.
Symptoms of low HGH testosterone levels after the age of thirty are not uncommon.

Here is an extensive list of common symptoms of low HGH /testosterone levels in both men and women:

Low Energy and Fatigue

Wrinkles (Loss of Skin Elasticity)

Diminished Sexual Drive & Desire

Weight Gain, particularly Hard-to-Lose Fat

Reduced Muscle Mass and Strength

Memory Loss

Decreased Motivation

Lack of Focus

Hair Loss

Increased Recovery Time from Wounds and Illness

High Cholesterol

Cellulite

Joint and Muscle Pain

Depression / Crankiness

Slower Metabolism

Osteoporosis

Sleep Disturbances

Headaches

If you experience any of the above symptoms low HGH/ testosterone levels, you do not have to worry. Aging is a myth! Every symptom can be reversed when you increase low HGH testosterone levels via HGH   testosterone therapy. HGH testosterone benefits are both physical and mental: including rejuvenation, fat loss, muscle building, sexual performance and more.

Below is another extensive list of some life-changing HGH testosterone benefits:

Fat Loss (even without diet and exercise)

Increased Strength, Energy and Stamina

Fast Muscle Growth and Recovery

Increased Flexibility

Increased Skin Elasticity (younger-looking, smoother skin)

Sharper Focus and Memory

Increased Motivation

Heightened Sense of well being, the zone feeling

Emotional Stability

Reduction of stress

Elimination of Depression (caused by low HGH Testosterone) & Fatigue

Renewed Sexual Drive & Desire

Improved Sexual Performance

Elimination of Erectile Dysfunction

Increased Sperm Production

Deeper, More Restful Sleep

Thicker Hair / Cessation of Hair Loss, Possible Hair Re-growth.

Sharper Eyesight

Reduced Cholesterol Levels

Reduction of Cellulite

Decrease in Muscle and Joint Pain

Increased Bone Density

Healthy metabolism

Healthier Heart Rate

Improved Immunity: including resistance to flu and colds.

Faster Healing of wounds and recovery from illness

Organ Growth (internal organs, including the brain, shrink with age).

Increased Red Blood Cell Production

Maintenance of Good Health, such as reducing risks of high blood pressure and heart attacks.

As you can see, the list is quite extensive and the benefits far outweigh the losses. Apart from improving the benefit of sexual desire, HGH even promotes the cognitive ability and increases muscle mass, thereby reducing fat. This is the hormone which restores as well as maintains youthful vigor and zeal that disappears slowly as men age.

Once released in the body, HGH stimulates the body parts naturally.

The result is an increase in the testicles production of more testosterone that in turn leads to increase in sexual desire as well as muscle mass. Now that I really got your attention, I am going to

introduce you to some top-quality effective HGH boosters in the next chapter.

Chapter 9

Natural HGH Booster L-Arginine and DHEA

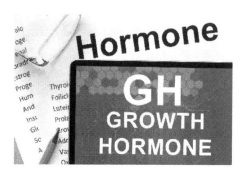

HGH is a complex molecule that is made up of more than 191 amino acids and one of the most important amino acids is L-arginine.

L-arginine is known to stimulate the production of HGH in your body. There are a lot of foods that contain this amino acid. The best sources include those such as lean meat, turkey, poultry, oatmeal, nuts, dark chocolate, beans etc. Including these foods in your diet is a must.

L-arginine is an amino acid that helps to increase the level of nitric oxide in blood. This ensures greater blood flow to the genitals. It helps men get harder and stiffer erections, while in women increased blood flow to the genitals can boosts libido and increase clitora sensitivity.

Some of the best supplements contain ingredients

such as 5HTP, GABA, Astragalus, Rhodiala Rosea and other important amino acids such as, l-valine, l-glutamine, l-tyrosine etc.,

A good quality supplement can contain up to 1000mg of amino acids per serving. This can be a great help in

stimulating the production of HGH. These supplements are usually considered safe and free of side effects. They do not have any sort of synthetic hormones in them. I personally take them on a regular basis and quite satisfied with the benefits they impart. Another big player men should consider before taking synthetic testosterone cream is DHEA.

Why is DHEA so important?

DHEA, dehydroepiandrosterone, is an adrenal steroid hormone in the body. It is made by the adrenal glands and converted to androgens, estrogens and other hormones. These are the hormones that regulate fat and mineral metabolism, sexual and reproductive function, and energy levels. DHEA levels increase until our mid to late 20's then gradually start to decline. DHEA production in the body may also decrease with the use of certain medications such as insulin and corticosteroids.

According to an article in the Journal of

Pharmacotherapy free testosterone levels begin to decline at a rate of 1% per year after age 40. It's estimated that 20% of men aged 60-80 years have levels below the lower limit of the norm.

DHEA, a precursor to testosterone, has been considered a significant nutrient to help support anabolic growth factors, increase muscle mass,

reduced body fat and sexual enhancement.

By the time your 65, your body only produces 10% of the DHEA that it produced when you were 20. That's why supplementation of DHEA is so vital for experiencing lower stress, staying healthier, and living longer.

What are the benefits of DHEA?

According to the Natural Medicines Comprehensive Database, DHEA is stated to be possibly effective for the following conditions:

Aging Skin – Taking DHEA orally seems to increase epidermal thickness, sebum production, skin hydration, and decrease facial skin pigmentation in elderly men and women

Erectile Dysfunction – Taking DHEA orally for 24 weeks seems to improve ED, orgasmic function, sexual desire and overall sexual satisfaction in men with erectile dysfunction. It may not be as beneficial in those with diabetes or neurological conditions.

Osteoporosis – Taking DHEA orally 50-100 mg per day seems to improve bone mineral density (BMD) in older women and men with osteoporosis or osteopenia.

DHEA is also thought to contribute to a sense of well-being when used by those with adrenal and/or

androgen insufficiency. In one placebo-controlled trial, DHEA supplementation for a 6- month period supported healthy physical and psychological outlook in men and women at ages 40-70 years. It may also support lean body mass in men and postmenopausal women. In another study, DHEA supplementation supported healthy male sexual function.

The caveat for taking DHEA should also be considered by men and women. If you are in good health free of diseases, DHEA may be the right choice you are searching for.

There are several different strengths of DHEA from 2 Mg, 5 Mg, 10 Mg, 25 Mg, 50 Mg and 100 Mg – always use the lowest dose appropriate for you.

What are the side effects of DHEA?

Possible side effects include hair loss, hair growth on the face (in women), aggressiveness, irritability and increased levels of estrogen. Calcium channel blockers may increase DHEA levels and supplementation should be avoided by those using calcium channel blockers. DHEA should not be used if pregnant or nursing, by those under the age of 18 or used by those with healthy levels of DHEA. Anyone with a history of hormone-related cancer should opt to avoid DHEA due to the probability of increased estrogen levels. Anyone with liver problems
or disease should avoid DHEA supplementation.
Because of the overwhelming evidence connecting low levels of DHEA to problems associated with aging the prudent use of DHEA can be a real game changer. Always consult with your doctor first.

Most of the research suggests that only people over age 35 should begin with DHEA therapy. For most people, the starting dose of DHEA is between 15–75 mg, taken in one daily dose. Many studies have shown promising results with use a daily dose of 50 mg.

Since almost everyone over age 35–40 has lower than optimal levels of DHEA, most people in this group should consider the benefits of supplementation and then test their blood DHEA levels later to make sure they are taking the proper dose. Normal serum reference ranges and ideal ranges of DHEA-S are:

	Normal (depending on age)	Ideal
Men	16.2-492 µg/dL	350-490 µg/Dl
Women	12-407 µg/dL	275-400 µg/dL

People over age 40 who do not supplement with DHEA usually have serum levels below 200 µg/dL, and many are below 100 µg/dL since a steady decline takes place after the third decade in life. There are different precautions for men and women that should be observed.

Before attempting to restore DHEA to youthful levels, men should know their serum PSA (prostate specific antigen) level. Men with prostate cancer or severe benign prostate disease are advised to avoid DHEA since it can be converted into testosterone and estrogen.

Therefore, men are advised to have a PSA and digital rectal exam before initiating DHEA to rule out existing prostate disease.

When taking DHEA we also recommend taking the following other nutrients daily:

Vitamin D	**5,000 – 10,000 IU**
Vitamin E (D-alpha tocopheryl succinate)	**400 IU**
Selenium	**200 mcg**
Gamma E Tocopherol with Sesame Lignans	**200 mg**
Lycopene Extract	**10 – 40 mg**
Boron	**3 – 10 mg**
Cruciferous Vegetable Extracts (as found in Triple Action Cruciferous Vegetable Extract)	**500 – 1000 mg**

It is important for men over 40 to have a physician check their PSA and DHEA-S serum levels every six to twelve months thereafter. Men should also periodically check their blood levels for free testosterone and estrogen to make sure that DHEA is following a youthful metabolic pathway.

Another key factor that affects testosterone and HGH levels in men is obesity.

Obesity and associated hyperinsulinemia suppress the action of lutenizing hormone (LH) in the testis, which can significantly reduce circulating testosterone levels (Mah and Wittert 2010), even in men under the age of 40 (Goncharov et al 2009). In addition, increased belly fat mass has been correlated with increased aromatase levels (Kalyani and Dobs 2007).

The vicious circle of low testosterone and obesity has been described as the hypogonadal/obesity cycle. In this cycle, a low testosterone level results in increased abdominal fat, which in turn leads to increased aromatase activity.

This enhances the conversion of testosterone to estrogens, which further reduces testosterone and increases the tendency toward abdominal fat (Cohen 1999, Tishova and Kalinchenko 2009).

In conclusion, men should be more cautious and do more research on balancing their testosterone. Never depend solely upon one test or one doctor's medical opinion.

In short, there appears to be an awful lot of men out there taking testosterone who probably shouldn't. Using hormones as a "cure-all" is a risky proposition, especially if your problems are related to lifestyle. What most men really need is a lifestyle change, in order to optimize their body's natural secretion of testosterone and other hormones

.

Frequently, I see commercials on TV upselling the merits of testosterone gel and how they can dramatically improve the quality of a man's sex life. These ads are paid endorsements that oversell and popularize a quick fix approach. In my opinion, the danger of introducing synthetic testosterone in a man's body outweighs the benefits. I can't help but reiterate using extreme caution and seeking out safer alternatives.

Negative Side Effects of Testosterone Gel

For a starter, testosterone gel or exogenous (non-natural) testosterone can cause stroke, heart attacks and increase risk of cancer. According to Drugs.com, this product may cause side effects including acne, headache, prostate disorder, emotional instability, hypertension and breast enlargement may increase the risk of developing an enlarged prostate, as well as prostate cancer. Those with liver disease, coronary disease, chest pain, high cholesterol, or a history of heart failure should consult with a doctor before taking testosterone. Diabetics might want to avoid its use too, as testosterone can affect blood sugar levels.

Long-term use of T gel products (more than a year or two) may contribute to liver disease and sleep apnea. Only your doctor can advise you as to how long you should use these products. Usage will vary based on the individual. Long term use of exogenous (non-natural) testosterone can also dampen the body's natural production of testosterone.

Taking testosterone over a extended period of time can cause peliosis hepatitis, a potentially fatal condition in which blood-filled cysts develop in the liver and/or kidneys. In men, testosterone can be converted to estrogen, sometimes resulting in gynecomastia (male breast enlargement), which may require surgery to correct.

Other Side Effects of Synthetic Testosterone

Testosterone can also cause jaundice (yellow skin), and alters cholesterol levels, which may lead to high blood pressure and heart disease. Users have also experienced difficult urination due to prostate enlargement, acne, greasy skin, edema (swelling of the feet and ankles), excitability, increased aggression, depression and headaches.

In many cases, the problem is not due to low T, but a more sinister like condition of what I call high E (high estrogen profile) vs low T.

High E (estrogen) is usually initiated by an unexpected culprit called xenoestrogens. This environmental nemesis is a real threat to male sexual health. Xenoestrogens are pervasive and lurk almost every where. A sexual warrior must not fall prey to this external enemy.

There are however alternative counter measures that can be taken by a proactive sexual warrior to ward off the negative onslaught of this enemy. A sexual warrior must protect and uphold his testosterone integrity. We will explore how to prevent the negative impact of xenoestrogens on male sexual health in the next chapter. Stay tuned because you don't want to miss this!

Testosterone Testing

If you are interested in testing your testosterone level then consider a saliva or urine test rather than a blood test. A saliva test can provide you with the best way to easily, accurately and inexpensively monitor your male hormone health. Urine tests are however more accurate. If you are 20-35 years of age it is best to be tested in the morning between 8–11am, since testosterone peaks at this time. Men who are age 40 or above can be tested at any time in the morning up until 2 pm for accuracy.

There are still several other advantages to salivary versus urine hormone assessments. The collection process is simple and painless. It's very easy to collect multiple samples of saliva/urine to determine your hormone levels throughout the course of a typical day. This is important since a man's testosterone levels can be as much as 40% higher in the morning than they are at night (the physiological reason for your morning erection). Testosterone levels can fluctuate daily. Multiple samples taken during a day can provide a more accurate profile of your testosterone level.

Salivary/urine hormone test kits are cost effective and time efficient. There is no need for waiting rooms, needles, paperwork, white coats or hassles.

Not only are they less expensive since sample collection can be done at home with results provided by e-mail. There are no additional payments, waiting time or follow up appointments which is the norm for most doctor's visits. All you need to do is collect your samples in the tubes provided in the test kit and mail them directly to the lab. Salivary samples are extremely stable and can be sent by regular mail with no problems.

Most importantly, it is essential to understand that inactive, blood-bound hormones do not filter into your saliva.

Salivary Hormone Test Kits (SHTK) provide the most accurate, physiological snapshot of your body's true hormonal potential because salivary testosterone tests measure the all-important free or bio-available hormones. Free or bio-available hormones are important because they act upon your cell receptor sites. In short, these tests check the form of testosterone that really counts.

Now let's compare SHTK to blood serum testosterone test.

First of all, blood serum assessments provide for a measurement of total testosterone only.

A total testosterone count includes both the free and bound forms of testosterone. The final results can be extremely misleading. Only one to three percent of the testosterone circulating in your blood is bio-available or capable of being used by your body. The other 97 to 99% is inactive and is bound to circulating proteins called SHBG or sex hormones binding globulin. These proteins prevent testosterone from binding with their target hormonal cellular receptors.

In other words, the testosterone is there, but nobody is at home to receive them. So quite often a man may have relatively normal levels of total testosterone but have drastically reduced levels of bio-available free testosterone.

So even though he has plenty of total testosterone in his blood he's still suffering all the brutal symptoms of low T.

Low T is not the same as true medical low T. So don't be duped or lured into thinking that there is a deeper problem when none exists. Men today are facing a real hormonal crisis that needs to be stopped! Testosterone levels in men on the average are 25% lower than they were just 20 years ago.

Estrogen levels have skyrocketed by as much as 40 percent! This assault on one's manhood is coming from several different directions. And the enemy is getting stronger and more powerful every day.

This is why, it's absolutely imperative that every man test his hormone status in order to find out exactly where he sits on the hormonal pyramid. If you're over the age of 30 chances are still very high that you **do** have elevated estrogen levels. If estrogen is up in your system testosterone is probably down. That's just the way it works.

Left unchecked the average man can sadly look forward to the following undesirable events:

Weaker Erections

Man Boobs

Diminished Sex drive

Shrunken Testicles

Muscle Replaced with Fat

Low Ejaculation Volume

I know this seems like quite a grim scenario to endure. The brutal combination of high estrogen and low testosterone can literally destroy a sexual warrior physically and emotionally. Fight back! Be the true sexual warrior within.

Page For Notes:

References:

http://EzineArticles.com/4733827

Read more:
http://www.ehow.com/about_5383047_dangers-testosterone.html#ixzz2uvS7VHP9

Read more:
http://www.ehow.com/about_5383047_dangers-testosterone.html#ixzz2uvRQHChO

Read more: What are the dangers of testosterone cream? | Answerbag
http://www.answerbag.com/q_view/1909107#ixzz2uvQUxpzJ

Read more: What are the dangers of testosterone cream? | Answerbag
http://www.answerbag.com/q_view/1909107#ixzz2uvQF2kN4
(Clinical Endocrinology: Nov 2007) - Salivary testosterone is a harmless and reliable marker of testosterone bio-availability. The results of this study support the inclusion of this bio-marker as a noninvasive approach in the evaluation of hormonal status.

(Psychoneuroendocrinology: Volume 10, Issue 1, 1985, Pages 77–81) - Changes in saliva testosterone after psychological stimulation in men.
(European Journal of Applied Physiology December 2001, Volume 86, Issue 2, pp 179-184 - Preliminary results on mood state, salivary testosterone:cortisol ratio and team performance in a professional soccer team.

Lund, BC, Bever-Stille KA, Perry PJ, "Testosterone and andropause: the feasibility of testosterone replacement therapy in elderly men." Pharmacotherapy, 1999 Aug; 19(8): 951-6.

2. The T-Factor: King of Hormones, Almark Publishing 2005 Pg 51

3. Baulieu EE. Thomas G, Legrain S, et al. Dehydroepiandrosterone (DHEA), DHEA sulfate, and aging: contribution of the DHEAge study to a sociobiomedical issue. Proc Natl Acad Sci USA. 2000;97 (8):4279-4284.

4. Broeder CE, Quindry MS, Brittingham K, et al. The Andro Project: Physiological and hormonal influences of androstenedione supplementation in men 35 to 65 years old participating in a high-intensity resistance

training program.

Arch Intern Med. 160:3093-3104

5. MacKenzie, , "How biorythms affect your life", Science Digest, 73,1973, 18 -22.

Chapter 10

The Testosterone Killer, Xenoestrogens High E or Low T?

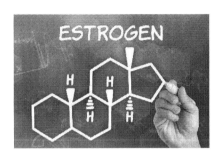

Fifty to one hundred years ago the average male testosterone level was around 1200 ng/deciliter. During that period, men were more driven, ambitious, aggressive, confident, courageous and pioneering. Today sexologist can see a drastic drop in T levels of men rendering them less masculine and more effeminate in nature. Over time as T levels dropped, estrogen levels rose thus creating a vicious downward spiral for the would be sexual warrior.

Estradiol is not a "female hormone" — it's something your body needs just as much as testosterone. In fact, some men who believe they're suffering from low testosterone may be suffering from low estradiol.

So, while it's important to make sure you have normal testosterone levels *for your body*, you also want to make sure you have normal estradiol levels as well.

Normal Estradiol Levels in Men

For men, normal ***total*** estradiol levels are somewhere between 20-55 pg/mL (2.0–5.5 ng/dL) and 10-40 pg/mL(1.0-4.0 ng/dL), depending on who you ask.

Men are gradually becoming less of a man each year! Due to the increased use of alcohol and estrogenic foods, environmental chemicals have triggered an increase production of estrogen in men. Chemicals in plastics may also play a factor in disrupting proper hormone function. Therefore, exposure to plastic chemicals have to be limited. For example, one should avoid the use of microwave food in plastic. Do not allow plastic water bottles to get too warm in the sun as the plastic estrogen base chemicals tend leach into the water.

It is this elevated estrogen level which will reduce the T/E ration and reduce the critical anabolic to catabolic ratio.

An ideal testosterone to estradiol level is 40 to 60 for an 30-40-year-old man as compared to a 20 yr. which would be 30-40. In assessing thousands of men via saliva testing, many of these tests find that less than 10% achieve these critical ratios and over 75% of them are less then 35 years old! Now that is sad! It is time for the warrior to wake up and map his battle strategy.

So, how do we fight back? Well to fight back, we must first identify who the enemy is outside of our bodies and how to neutralize that threat. We will address how the enemy is able to impact our health shortly. Our first mission leads us to a culprit called xenoestrogens. Men everywhere must garner their shields and learn to seek and destroy xenoestrogens to win back their captured masculine glory.

As men get older, their testosterone level gradually decline typically about 1 percent a year after age 30.
Testosterone levels peak at around age 20, then they begin a steadily fall. By the time men hit 60 their testosterone levels are 1/3 of what they had in their 20s.
By the time men are 80, they have 20 percent of what they had in their youth. No wonder it seems like your manhood is just slipping away. OK, that's bad enough. But what many men fail to realize is that things can get

much worse.
Xenoestrogens are "alien-estrogens" that are not made in your body. The word xenoestrogen is derived from the Greek words ξένο (xeno, meaning foreign), οἶστρος

(estrus, meaning sexual drive) and γόνο (gene, meaning "to generate") and literally means "foreign estrogen". Xenoestrogens are also called "environmental hormones" or endocrine disrupting compounds (EDC). Most scientists that study xenoestrogens, including The Endocrine Society, regard them as serious environmental chemical hazards that have hormone disruptive effects on both wildlife and humans.

Today both men and women tend to suffer from estrogen dominance or having too much estrogen and a lesser balance of other sex hormones. There is simply too much of it around and it is impossible to fully escape its impact. Plastics, car exhaust, pesticides, meats, soaps,

carpet, furniture, and paneling are just some examples of xeno sources. On-and-off sinus problems, headaches, dry eyes, asthma, cold hands and feet, and may also be attributed to your exposure to xenoestrogens.

Over time, xenoestrogens exposure can cause more chronic problems such as arthritis, and gallbladder disease.

The problem of xenoestrogens is so pervasive in our modern society. External estrogen should at all cost be

avoided. The best place to start is in your own home. Here are some common recommendations:

Throw away all pesticides, herbicides, and fungicides.

- Throw away cosmetics that have toxic ingredients and switch to organic and "clean" cosmetics.

- Throw away nail polish and nail polish removers.

- Use organic soaps and toothpastes.

- Don't use fabric softeners as it puts petrochemical right on your skin.

- Use only naturally based perfumes. Most perfumes are   petro-chemical based.

Have a good water filter for your source of water.

- Limit the use of plastic goods since all plastic leach into the environment.

- Eat only organic based whole foods.

- Avoid surfactants found in many condoms and diaphragm gels.

- New carpet can give off noxious fumes.

- Be aware of noxious gas such as that from copiers and printers, carpets, fiberboards and computer monitors that emit high level of electromagnetic force (EMF).

- Avoid X-rays as much as possible.

- Do not microwave food in plastic containers, and especially avoid the use of plastic wrap to cover food for microwaving.

- Wash your food well to rid the pesticides. Bathe food in water that contains vinegar and lemon juice for 20 minutes before cooking.

Be aware of chronic stress leading to adrenal fatigue, another leading cause of progesterone depletion and thus estrogen dominance. Balancing excessive estrogen requires taking into consideration steps to reduce and remove stressors which compromise adrenal function. As mentioned in my previous chapter, adrenal glands play a crucial role in the production of testosterone and must not be compromised. After all, a man needs all the testosterone he can produce in a healthy manner.

Fortification of the adrenal hormone androgen via supplementation of DHEA can be quite effective. If you live in an industrialized country, there may well be more than 100,000 different environmental estrogens or xenoestrogens that challenge your health & well-being.

These harmful chemicals must be identified and avoided, as they have been shown to cause birth defects, abnormal sexual development, problems with the nervous system, the immune system, cancer, PMS/PMT, infertility, osteoporosis.

If you eat meat and dairy products in harmony with your blood type, it is imperative that the label states: "No added hormones; no antibiotics, no pesticides", otherwise you will be adding fuel to a fire that will hurt you.

Petroleum derivatives also called petro-chemicals, are found in most personal care products and commercially grown meat and dairy. BPA, PCB's and phthalates, are universally recognized as exerting an estrogenic effect on humans. Prescription hormones, such as ethynyl estradiol are also foreign to the human body.

Since the list of commercial petroleum compounds (petro chemicals) are so extensive (>100,000. Under this category are the following common products.

Xeno-estrogen List of Products to Avoid
Mineral Oil
Soaps

Lotions

Shampoos

Cosmetics

Fragrances: perfumes, room fresheners

House Hold Cleaners

Pesticides

Plastics: (never microwave)

Detergents

Preservatives

Artificial Sweeteners

Pharmaceutical Drugs

Consider going on the offense by being a sexual warrior. A diet designed to purify the body with foods that promote detoxification will help restore a healthy balance of hormones and the body's circadian rhythms.

Studies that have been conducted in people who ate a diet rich in cruciferous vegetables such as, kale, collards, cabbage, brussels sprouts, broccoli, & radishes versus those who did not eat such foods. The cruciferous group decreased their odds of forming cancer in the body by approximately 50%! There is no known pharmaceutical drug that can match this prevention level. These cruciferous vegetables are known to contain special compounds such as indole 3 carbinol that change a dangerous cancer-causing form of estrogen into a benign protective form.

Testosterone levels for the general male population have declined steadily for most men of varied ages as early as 1940. Many serious health problems began to rise after 1940; when we started using DDT, chemical pesticides, petrochemicals, synthetic hormones and plastics.

"Low- T" used to be thought of as a problem for men 60 or older. It is now appearing in men as young as 30! I believe part of the problem is the result of stress, pollution from toxins, heavy metals and of course the infamous xenoestrogens.

We now know that the natural role of estrogen in a male is to provide bio-feedback to the pituitary gland and regulate testicular testosterone production. The xenoestrogens do the same thing, but their levels are not regulated. They are often more powerful than the real estrogen we make in our own body. These alien rouge estrogens can shut off male testosterone production prematurely, leading to low T and low luteinizing hormones. The problem is not an issue that he cannot make his own testosterone but rather the failure of his pituitary gland to signal the testicle to make it.

Such an outcome can be attributed to xenoestrogen effects as well as pituitary damage.

Some of my "Low-T" male clients don't really need more testosterone. They just need to get the xenoestrogens out of their system.

In women, xenoestrogens stimulate estrogen-sensitive tissues excessively, leading to diseases like breast fibrocystic disease, endometriosis, heavy menses with breakthrough bleeding, uterine fibroids, PMS, breast and uterine cancer.

The first course of action should start with your food choices. Strive to eat only organic vegetables and grass-fed organic meats. Non-organic foods are coated with pesticides and herbicides and the animals are injected with xenoestrogens growth compounds to make them gain weight faster. Another good precaution is the avoidance of farm-raised salmon. Many of them often contain unsafe levels of PCBs and pesticides that are xenoestrogen in origin.

Avoid all non- organic dairy products. These dairy products (milk, cheese, or ice cream) are made by pregnant cows or goats full of growth hormones. A healthier alternative to consuming regular milk is almond, rice or coconut milk. Regular cow milk acts on your body just as human estrogens. You can get about 20 different kinds of cow or goat hormones with each glass of milk or piece of cheese.

It is clear from medical research that the incidence of breast, ovarian, prostate, and other cancers are linked to the consumption of dairy products.

Xenoestrogens and growth hormones are often found in commercial milk and milk products. Traces of these compounds can even be found in some organic milk. I always advise my clients to avoid dairy at all cost. Milk in general is good food for a calf, but not a human being.

Again, try to avoid the use of plastic whenever possible. Plastics, are commonly formulated with chemicals that act a lot like estrogen. When you inhale that new car odor and notice the smell of new shower curtains or new synthetic carpet, you have already been exposed to xenoestrogens. Using food wrapped in saran wrap, drinking from Styrofoam cups, and synthetic cleaners all allow xenoestrogens to enter your body. Even cosmetics contain xenoestrogens called phthalates and parabens. If you want to get rid of xenoestrogens, work hard to eliminate plastics.

Opt to use natural home-construction materials such as stone, tile, wood, and non-toxic paints. Use a glass shower door rather than a shower curtain. Filter the water in your home either with a whole house filter or at the tap using an over the counter filter. The use of shower filters are also recommended. Drink from paper cups or better yet, glass or ceramic.

Avoid eating canned foods as they are sometimes lined with plastic inside.

Cook with glass or metal pots; never use Teflon or non-stick coating as they off gas toxins into your food when heated. Filter your water with a charcoal filter attached to your tap. The Pure Water Filter is an inexpensive good start. Carry water in a metal flask rather than a plastic container. Avoid using chemical pesticides and lawn chemicals. Find a "green" company to help you with pests and landscaping while making sure they are using products that have no xenoestrogens in them.

For construction projects, make sure they are not using chemical adhesives, insulation, vinyl siding, vinyl windows, chemical paints, solvents, sealants or other plastic compounds to save time and money. These products contain xenoestrogens that will leak into your home for years to come. Spend the money up front to build your home with the techniques that are now available to make your home "green" but also non-toxic.

Young children tend to spend lots of time on the floor at home. Unfortunately, this is also the period when the worst exposure can occur.

Here is a good website to check out on finding more ways to remove xenoestrogens and toxins from your body and home.

www.everydayexposures.com

References:

1. Fisch, Harry; and Golden, Robert,
Topic 3.16: Environmental estrogens and sperm
counts.
Pure Appl. Chem., 2003.
75 (11 -12): p. 2181-2193.

2. Matthiessen, Peter,
Topic 4.1: Historical perspective on endocrine disruption
in wildlife.
Pure Appl. Chem., 2003.
75 (11 -12): p. 2197-2206.
3. Guillette, L.J.J.a.I., Taisen,
Topic 4.7: Contaminant-induced endocrine and
reproductive
alterations in reptiles.
Pure Appl. Chem., 2003.
75 (11 -12): p. 2275-2286.
4. Sumpter, John P.,
Endocrine Disrupters in the Aquatic
Environment: An Overview.
Acta
hydrochimica et hydrobiologica, 2005.
33 (1): p. 9-16.
5. Harvey, Philip W. and Everett, David J.,

Regulation of endocrine-disrupting chemicals:
Critical overview and deficiencies in toxicology and risk
assessment for human health.
Best Practice & Research Clinical Endocrinology &
Metabolism, 2006. 20 (1): p. 145- 165

Chapter 11

The Testosterone Diet/Food for Sex

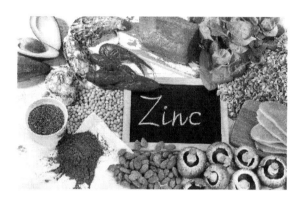

Before delving into specific diets or foods that are beneficial to the reproductive system and optimal testosterone levels, I would like to first share with you a more ancient perspective on sex. What is the purpose of sex? While sex is obviously necessary for procreation of the species, it too can lead to the re-creation of our selves. Modern men usually view sex as a means of defining their masculinity, self validation or simply as a recreational reward after a period of stress. For couples, intimacy involving sex usually triggers the release of a hormone called oxytocin or the bonding hormone.

The release of the hormone oxytocin often forges a deep emotional connective bond between couples. This bonding process is necessary to motivate couples to stay together long enough and commit to a relationship. If a woman is not having an orgasm, then she is not experiencing the bonding effect of oxytocin. Giving a woman an orgasm is one of the best assurances that she stays connected to you. All sexual warriors should make sure that their woman is well satisfied before having their own orgasm.

Sex is not necessarily a function that must be performed on a regular basis such as eating to stay alive. The organs that control reproduction glands are more efficient and potent when given a period of rest. As I mentioned in one of my previous chapters, men should not try to be a superman or porno star in the bedroom. Performance anxiety can lead to quite the opposite results that most men want.

Media hype leading to over-stimulation and obsession of the mind with sexual ideations and fantasies are usually the common causes. Exposure to pornographic magazines and films on a regular basis can either boost or desensitize a man's arousal mechanism. If not checked, higher and higher levels of stimulation will be needed for a man to achieve an optimal level of arousal leading to an erection.

Abstaining from sex for a minimum period of 6 weeks or 1-3 months while cultivating one's health can serve as a good strategy to cure virtually most cases of non-medical impotency. Emphasis should be placed upon the cultivation of sexual fluids, avoiding the indiscriminate loss of semen and improve blood circulation. Decreasing stress and exposure to environmental xenoestrogens is always advisable.

Both man and primates are the only animals that nature allows for the sex act to be performed at will. All other animals have definite mating periods and are driven to procreate by nature. The act of reproduction is primarily a sacrifice or catabolic process throughout the animal and plant kingdom. The term catabolic refers to the break down of tissue or energy because of stress. When something is lost or gained.

Reproduction is a movement towards depletion and in some cases death. After a plant bears fruit, it is often weakened and in some cases, dies due to the huge loss of life force needed for reproduction. The reproductive function in humans depends upon the tonification of the kidney yang function as documented in Chinese Medicine.

Understanding and managing the kidney yang function can prove to be a major player in improving testosterone levels and male erectile dysfunction. Exactly what is kidney yang? If there is a yang then there must be a yin. According to Chinese traditional medicine, the kidneys represent the primal energy source and pilot light of the body.

The kidney organ system represents the fundamental root of all yin and yang energy of the body. The kidney energy system also stores the body's essence referred to as jing. This substance or essence must be maintained in order to age well and live long with mental clarity. Maintaining healthy kidney energy is necessary for both healthy aging and optimal sexual function.

In traditional Chinese Medicine (TCM), some of the symptoms of kidney yang deficiency are frequent urination, difficulty urinating, and edema. The adrenal gland function is also tied into the yang aspect of the kidneys. This is why some of the symptoms of kidney yang deficiency are cold limbs, lack of energy and sexual dysfunction. Temperature, energy, and sexual function are all regulated in part by the adrenal hormones.

Chinese Medicine considers the male and female sexual function, including the condition of the sperm and egg to be associated with the kidney function.

For example, in my clinic, I realized that many people who suffered from infertility issues may also have their kidney yin or yang out of balance. This imbalance can easily affect the quality of their egg or sperm. The preferred treatment plan is to tonify the kidneys. Balancing the kidney yin and yang function can improve most sexual issues such as impotence and lowered libido. Beware that having sex too infrequently can also cause a depletion of yang energy.

The kidney yin energy is for increasing flexibility, decreasing inflammation, hormonal balance and rejuvenation of the adrenal glands and body in general. Stress can disrupt and deplete the kidney energy. Kidney yin tonics are often prescribed by Chinese doctors to their patients to offset the damage caused by stress and protect the function of the kidney yang energy.

Now that you have a basic understanding why kidney yang energy is so important let us continue with diet. A testosterone diet plan should incorporate the use of specific foods and herbs that will target and increase the kidney energy (qi) and ultimately raw sexual energy.

According to Chinese Medicine engaging in regular sex can benefit the internal organs and balance the yin and the yang of the body. However, over-doing it can affect the kidney essence for both the men and the women. Frequent ejaculation in men tends to exhaust the reproductive essence stored in the kidneys. This essence is often referred to as Jing by the Chinese.

Jing is easily replaced by young men but becomes harder to replace as men age and vital energy declines. This is why, the ancient Taoist practiced methods of sexual conservation to replenish the Jing and promote longevity. Appropriate regularity of sex is subjective and can vary from person to person depending on age, constitution, health, diet, lifestyle and even the season.

According to Traditional Chinese Medicine TCM, the following foods are considered suitable for kidney support: scallops, small dried prawns, walnuts, chives, goji berries, black beans, lamb or lamb bone soup, beef or beef bone soup.

Excessive physical activity can also cause a disruption to your yang energy. Moderate amounts of walking daily between 30 minutes to an hour in a peaceful natural setting can promote a healthy flow of yang in your kidneys.

How does kidney yin energy affect a man's sexual health? Kidney Yang Deficiency can cause low back pain, erectile dysfunction, prostate problems frequent urination and adrenal fatigue. These problems should be addressed before considering the use of testosterone boosters or low T gel.

A note of caution commercially raised cattle and chickens in the United States are routinely injected with various growth hormones.   These injected hormones are banned in the European Union and a multitude of other nations due to their potentially carcinogenic properties. Some of these growth hormones act very similarly to endocrine disruptors in the body, skewing hormones and paving the way for a variety of cancers. Additionally, commercially raised cattle are given antibiotics on a routine basis and fed cheap feeds that are largely based on genetically modified corn. Any form of food that is considered an endocrine disrupter should be avoided by both men and women.

A well-balanced testosterone diet favors the use of natural organic selections tempered to satisfy the nutritional needs of the individual.

A kidney yang diet can be highly beneficial to men provided they do not have an excess of kidney yang energy.

According to the 5-element theory, a balance of yin and yang energy in the body should be considered first before trying to rev up the body to a hyper yang state in order to be sexually active.

Yang represents the energy that is responsible for warming and activating bodily functions. When this energy is depleted your body begins to slow down, displaying signs of under activity and sensations of coldness. On the following page, I have provided a list of foods and categories that can help build deficient sexual energy. These foods are highly nutritious for the male reproductive system.

Foods to tonify qi and blood to a yang energy state are listed below:

Grains	Quinoa, black rice, wheat germ
Vegetables	Leek, mustard greens, onion, radish, scallion, squash, sweet potato, turnip, watercress, beets
Fruit	Cherry, lychee, logan, peach, raspberry, strawberry
Nuts and seeds	Chestnuts, pine nuts, pistachio nuts, walnuts
Fish	Anchovy, lobster, mussel, prawn, shrimp, trout, sardines
Meat	Chicken, lamb, venison, kidneys (both beef and lamb)
Herbs and spices	Basil, black pepper, caper, cayenne, chive seed, cinnamon bark, clove, dill seed, fennel seed, fenugreek seed, garlic, ginger, horseradish, nutmeg, peppermint, rosemary, sage, savory, spearmint, star anise, turmeric, thyme, white pepper
Beverages	Chai tea, jasmine tea
Supplements	Algae, ginseng (American, Chinese, and Korean), pine pollen, royal jelly

Examples of common western foods that can be used to build yang energy are:

Mussels cooked with a little garlic

Roast chicken with sage and thyme

Roasted vegetables with rosemary

Rice porridge with cinnamon, nutmeg and a little brown sugar

Leek and potato soup with black pepper

The above listed spices should be used frequently. When it comes to cooking, the saying goes "the spicier the better."

It is our basic diet that plays a critical role in our sexual health. First of all, if you're overweight, research shows that simply shedding excess pounds may increase your testosterone levels by reducing estrogen receptor sites in the body.

A sexual warrior should be warned that testosterone levels can decrease after you eat sugar. This is likely because sugar and fructose raises your insulin level, which is another factor leading to low testosterone. Ideally, keep your total fructose consumption below 25 grams per day. If you have insulin resistance and are overweight, have high blood pressure, diabetes, or high cholesterol, you'd be well advised to keep it under 15 grams per day. Research shows that a diet with less than

40 percent of energy from fat (mainly from animal sources, i.e. saturated) leads to a decrease in testosterone levels. So, fats is where it's at. It is very important to use the right kinds and amounts of fat in your diet.

I also urge you to think of foods as medicine rather than just for calories. Food should not be used solely for comfort. Food is not meant to make you feel good or perk you up when you're lonely and sad. It should not be used solely to cheer you up when your boss is mean and nasty and the wife and kids are mad at you. Using food for comfort is just as bad as drinking alcohol when you are depressed. Both can wreak havoc on your health.

It is a well-known fact that vegetables can have a positive clinical effect on the body. Broccoli, for example, can lower the bad estrogen because it is a cruciferous vegetable. Many foods, such as pomegranates, walnuts and cacao, will cause your arteries to dilate and pump out precious nitric oxide to aid blood flow to your penis. The high testosterone diet is yet another example of how foods can be used to raise total testosterone levels. Monounsaturated and saturated fats can help boost testosterone levels. Some good examples of these include red meat, whole fat dairy products, avocados, nuts, seeds, olive oil and flax oil.

The hormone testosterone is present in the male and female body. It is more dominant in men and the primary male sex hormone. It also serves many other purposes such as bone formation, muscle strength, energy and mood regulation. When testosterone levels are low, social life, fitness level and mental capacity can be negatively impacted. Many times, men look for a boost from supplements, creams and injections to increase their levels of testosterone. These approaches are often accompanied with side effects. Food is a much safer and more affordable option.

As men age, testosterone naturally declines. This decline can lead to muscle wasting and an increase of fat on the body. It is testosterone that causes a decline in fat cells and the building of lean metabolically active muscles. These muscles in turn can keep weight stabilized and reduce the risk factors for diseases. That is why it is important to have a normal amount of testosterone in the body.

Fats

Under normal circumstances, fat is often viewed as the nemesis to health. Although that might be true, there is a whole other side to fats that actually offer some benefits to the body. There are good fats and bad ones. Monounsaturated and saturated fats can help boost testosterone levels. Some healthy examples of foods derived from fats can include red hormone free range meats, whole fat organic dairy products, avocados, nuts, seeds, olive, coconut and flax oil.

Cruciferous Vegetables

Estrogen is a hormone that can inhibit the release of testosterone in the system. A great way to counter excess estrogen is by eating cruciferous vegetables. They often contain compounds called indoles which help keep testosterone production high and estrogen low. Other examples of these vegetables are brussels sprouts, cabbage, broccoli and cauliflower.

Eggs

Eggs are one of the main sources of protein for athletes. Eggs are high in B-vitamins as well as omega 3. The best eggs to eat should be caged free and pasteurized. One other aspect of eggs is the fact that they contain cholesterol, which can actually help boost testosterone levels.

Vitamin Rich Foods

As a side benefit to eating foods that boost testosterone, you may also notice an increase in your sex drive and sperm count. B-vitamins, vitamin-E and zinc are the key nutrients that cause this increase in testosterone levels.

Examples of foods that contain these vitamins and supports healthy testosterone levels are asparagus, raw oysters, bananas, brown rice and pine nuts.

Research shows that consuming more protein than carbs may lower testosterone levels. Protein should comprise of no more than 20-30% of our diet. Do not exceed the bodybuilding standard of 1 gram of protein per pound of bodyweight per day. Make sure most of your protein comes from animal sources or high protein vegetables such as beans. Vegetarian diets that are low in fat and quality protein are associated with lower testosterone levels in males for that group.

Monounsaturated Fats

Concentrate on choosing monounsaturated fats found in nuts, olives, olive oil and avocados, and saturated fats from hormone free meats and egg yolks. Unorthodox as this advice may be, research suggests that polyunsaturated fats lower testosterone levels, while monounsaturated and even saturated fats raise T levels. Research suggests that when total fat, saturated fat and monounsaturated fat intake increase, so does testosterone. Coconut Fat (MCT) are ideal for increasing energy and raising testosterone. Red meats and dairy products (not the fat-free varieties) are also a good source of protein and saturated fat. Worried about your heart health? Research states that most saturated fat found in beef, chicken and

pork does not raise LDL ("bad") cholesterol levels. Eating modest proportions of meat with ample vegetables can strike a healthy balance.

Vegetables

Eat plenty of cruciferous vegetables like broccoli, cauliflower, celery, brussel sprouts, cabbage, arugula, watercress, bok choy, turnip greens, collard greens, rutabaga, radishes, daikon, kohlrabi and kale. All of these vegetables have phyto-chemicals that can lower bad estrogens and potentially lessen their negative impact on testosterone levels.

Alcohol

Alcohol can have positive health benefits but too much can lower T levels. Stay under a few glasses of red wine per week. Try to avoid beer. Beers tends to lower testosterone levels due to one of its key estrogenic ingredient, hops.

Meats

Studies show that vegetarian diets can lead to lower blood testosterone levels and higher amounts of "inactive" testosterone even when protein intake is the same. Be sure to consume organic versions of poultry, beef, fish (wild caught) and pork.

Red meat is particularly good in moderation due to its higher levels of saturated fat and zinc. Zinc is a mineral associated with higher T levels. Consuming more protein than carbs can increase the loss of testosterone through urination. Protein is necessary for higher testosterone levels but too much can have a negative impact on the kidneys.

The following dietary characteristics were associated with relatively low testosterone levels among the male subjects studies:

Percentage of fat in the diet

Saturated fat intake per unit body weight

Monounsaturated fat intake per unit body weight

Protein intake as a percent of diet

The studies showed that a diet high in fat promoted increased testosterone but was bad for a man's heart. Maintaining a 2:1 ratio of carbohydrates to protein intake can boost T levels as compared to men taking in high levels of protein to build muscles. There appears to be a conflict of health when comparing a diet that promotes testosterone production vs one that promotes longevity.

Men who consume a moderate amount of protein need not worry about T production levels dropping.

A daily protein intake of 1 gram per kilogram of body weight can supply plenty of protein for muscle growth and repair without risking suppression of testosterone production.

What about the positive effect of saturated fat intake on testosterone levels? Is it worth risking heart health? It is not necessary for men to load up on fatty meats, full-fat dairy products, or tropical oils in order to maximize their testosterone levels. Stay away from foods that contain trans-fat.

 Liberal use of olive oil in cooking will provide plenty of monounsaturated fat. A diet high in this beneficial fat also promotes a healthy HDL cholesterol level which helps to prevent heart disease. On the other hand, a high saturated-fat diet without adequate vegetables and fruit can lead to arterial disease and indirectly cause erectile dysfunction by reducing blood flow to the penis.

In summary, here are some of the best recommendations based on clinical research that can have a positive impact on testosterone levels as it relates to food.

Protein

Eat adequate but not excessive amounts of protein. Eight ounces of meat per day as well as some low fat or fat-free dairy products will provide a healthy quantity of protein. Organic whey protein concentrate powder can also be utilized to supplement one's diet. If you want to use a dietary analysis computer program, limit daily protein intake to 1 gram per kilogram of body weight. Avoid consuming more than 30 grams of protein per meal. The excess protein will turn into fat if left unchecked.

Use olive oil regularly.

This provides plenty of monounsaturated fats that promote testosterone but contain low levels of the polyunsaturated fats. I prefer to use the cold press extra virgin oil brands and avoid oils like sunflower or canola oils. Coconut oil however, is always good with many additional health benefits due to its medium chain triglycerides content or (MCT) in coconut = pure energy-conversion to fat. Wow! Avoid most other vegetable oils because they contain high levels of the polyunsaturated fats that are associated with lower testosterone levels.

Eat whole fruits and vegetables but avoid extra fiber supplements. There is too much evidence that fruits and vegetables are beneficial to the health. Never try to avoid them to maximize your testosterone level. It is also a good idea to read food labels and avoid cereals and other products that add bran or other fiber. Natural whole grains are fine.

Make healthy carbohydrates an important part of your diet. A moderate amount of pasta, rice, and/or bread with meals will keep your carbohydrate-to-protein ratio at testosterone-promoting levels. It will also build a level of stored-carbohydrate (glycogen) in your muscles that will keep your energy level high and give you plenty of endurance for sports activities.

Maintain a healthy body weight

Body mass index is negatively associated with lower testosterone levels. The heavier you are for your height or being overweight can create extra estrogen receptor cellular sites that convert healthy testosterone to estrogen. Pinching the fat around your midsection is a quick and handy method of determining if you carry too much body fat.

Eating according to the seasons and one's constitutional body type is key to preserving and maintaining health. For more in depth information on this subject see Chinese Medicine (Henry Liu, Chinese System of Food Cure1986).

The Chinese system of food stresses avoiding an unbalanced diet of uncooked or raw foods that can have a cooling effect on the body. A man's sexual libido is usually the result of yang heat energy generated by the kidney qi energy or the pilot light of his body. Foods can be classified as having thermogenic properties (warming), energetic actions and flavor attributes markers for determining how they impact the body.

This approach is based upon what is known as the 5 element theory of health.

The elements are identified to represent earth, wood, fire, water, metal and are associated with the 5-yin internal organ system. Wood is associated with the liver/gallbladder and fire is associated with the heart and small intestine system. Energy can either be hot, cold, cooling or warming in nature.

The taste or flavor of a food can be classified as salty, sour, bitter, sweet or pungent.

For example, wood type foods are sour in taste as compared to earth type foods which are sweet to the taste. Low libido, cold hands or feet, and frequent urination are signs that can indicate a yang deficiency state of a person. In order to cure this type of problem, a diet with yang type foods are recommended to increase the warmth and qi of the body. Both herbs and exercises may also be prescribed by a Chinese doctor to balance any deficiency noted. You are not what you eat but what you digest or assimilate.

Try the "Mediterranean Diet" for a natural boost of nitric oxide as well. Increase your intake of lean proteins, dark leafy vegetables like spinach and kale. Increase also the consumption of dairy and nuts. Try eating more watermelon when in season and beets to boost citrulline and arginine levels of the body.

A list of some potent
Nitric oxide (NO) boosting foods should include:
Nuts like almonds, pecans, walnuts, as well as pine nuts can increase nitric oxide.
Meat including beef, pork and chicken and liver are especially high in citrulline.
Salmon, trout, tilapia and especially cold-water fish like tuna increases nitric oxide levels in the body.

Dark leafy green vegetables like spinach, collard greens beets and beet root are also beneficial.

Fruit like watermelon contains both arginine and citrulline. Most of the citrulline is in the rind.

Onions and garlic also both contain arginine and citrulline.

Legumes like beans, lentils, and peanuts increase blood flow.

Dark Chocolate, with at least 70% cacao is also very beneficial. Stay away from milk chocolate which is loaded with sugar and fat.

Intermittent Interval Fasting or IIF is another useful modality that every sexual warrior should utilize to facilitate raising testosterone levels and improving sexual performance. **IIF** describes a dietary modality with cycles between a period of fasting and non-fasting. In some context, fasting allows for the consumption of a limited number of low-calorie beverages such as coffee or tea. Although research studies do not show a direct correlation to increasing testosterone levels, there is evidence to support an increase via HGH. An increase in HGH levels are usually associated with increases in fitness potential, cellular regeneration, shortening of muscle recovery and improve blood flow. Improved blood flow can upgrade erectile dysfunction and boost a man's libido to a higher degree. Intermittent fasting acts to turn on certain genetic repair mechanisms that enhance cellular rejuvenation.

Researchers at the Intermountain Medical Center Heart Institute found that men, who had fasted for 24 hours, had a 2000% increase in circulating HGH. Women who were tested had a 1300% increase in HGH. The researchers found that the fasting individuals had significantly reduced their triglycerides, boosted their HDL cholesterol and stabilized their blood sugar.

The best way to begin fasting is by giving your body 12 hours between dinner and breakfast every single day. This allows 4 hours to complete digestion and 8 hours for the liver to complete its detoxification cycle.

 Allow this habit to become a standard part of your lifestyle, try taking one day a week and extending the fast to 14-18 hours. Eventually, you may choose to do a full 24 hours fast once a week.

Food Abstinence and Sex

A sexual warrior should also learn how to abstain from gorging on a big meal prior to having sex. After consuming a large meal, the body has to work hard at digesting and assimilating the nutrients in foods. When one calculates the amount of energy expenditure used by the digestive system, it is almost comparable to walking a brisk mile.

Most people are already keenly aware of how they tend to feel sluggish after eating a large meal and sometimes even a modest one. When it comes to having great sex a warrior needs all the energy he or she can muster. In terms of blood flow, most of the body's blood supply becomes accumulated in the stomach area during the process of digestion. This can cause a decline in peripheral blood flow to the limbs and penis. After a large meal, it is advisable to allow more time for digestion before engaging in sex.

In other words, less blood flow can easily cause a weaker erection if most of the blood is still in the abdomen. Based upon my experiences and those of others, I would strongly suggest that a sexual warrior wait at least a minimum of 2 hours and an optimal period of 4 hours after a meal before engaging in sex. Drinking liquids are ok as longs as they are low in sugar and contain no phosphoric acid. Commercial sodas are usually high in sugar and phosphoric acid.

References:

1. What science says about intermittent fasting by Dr. Mercola June 28, 2013

2. Hurley, B.F., Seals, D.R., Hagberg, J.M., Goldberg, A.C., Ostrove, S.M., Holloszy, J.O., Wiest, W.G., Goldberg, A.P. (1984). High-density-lipoprotien cholesterol in bodybuilders v powerlifters, negative effects of androgen use. JAMA, 252(4), 507-513.

3. Kleiner, S.M. (1991). Performance-enhancing aids in sports, health consequences and nutritional alternatives. J Am Coll Nutr, 10(2), 163-76.

4. Kleiner, S.M., Bazzarre, T.L., Litchford, M.D., (1990). Metabolic profiles, diet, and health practices of championship male and female bodybuilders. J Am Diet Assoc, 90(7), 962-967.

5. Chinese Medicine (Henry Liu), Chinese System of Food Cure1986)

6. Testosterone and cortisol in relationship to dietary nutrients and resistance exercise" by Volek, Kraemer,Bush, Incledon, and Boetes of Penn State University, was published in the Journal of Applied Physiology, volume 82, pages 49-54.ine.

Chapter 12

TESTOSTERONE BOOSTERS AND SUPPLEMENTATION

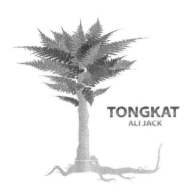

Natural Testosterone Boosters and Supplementation

Sexual union is such a wonderful gift given to mankind. Many creatures in the animal kingdom are not endowed with this opportunity, emotions and freedom of choice when it comes to engaging in sex. Animals in general, are quite limited when making choices and operate primarily on the basis of an instinctual mating season. Most sexual encounters between them are usually brief and unemotional in nature, serving only the need to procreate. For most people sex is about forming relationships. Question, what do I do when the thrill is gone or almost gone? How do I avoid being an old man wishing for younger days?

I will answer these questions soon enough. But first make an affirmation to yourself that sex is worth fighting for. Unlike most men, there is a constant battle within and without between estrogen dominance and testosterone supremacy. When it comes to testosterone survival, there is no surrender.

What is the best approach for men to take to improve their sex life? Well the answer should surprise you. There is none. One shoe does not fit all. Each man represents a unique constellation of needs, body chemistry and desires. The right equation or formulation of supplements depends on a variety of factors such as age, fitness level, diet, environmental exposure to xenoestrogens and psychological profile. After carefully reviewing many sex-pill formulations on the market, I discovered a necessary combination that must be present to achieve results.

The key ingredients should include a custom mix of testosterone precursors (stimulates the production of testosterone in the body), estrogen blockers, the brain neurotransmitter dopamine and at least one vasodilator to boost nitric oxide. I will discuss in detail the importance of nitric oxide later.

A more enlightened approach should focus more on the principles of a good individualized testosterone supplementation program. The most important guiding principles are selection, stacking, negative feedback loop, cycling and daily rotation of supplements. What will work for today may not work the next week or month.

This is the point of frustration when many men get discouraged and simply surrender to mediocrity.

Ok, let's get started on selection. Selection is a process of deciding what's best for you.

Based upon my own personal experiences and those of my clients, a good starting point should entail the use of vitamin C, 1-3 grams daily, selenium 100mcg, zinc 50mg followed up with adaptogens. Testosterone boosters should be used by men 40 or above since the average rate of testosterone decline is greater than previous years. Young men of 18 years of age should use adaptogens rather than testosterone boosters because they are already at their peak production. Adaptogens can still be used by men over 40.

What are adaptogens and how do they benefit us?
An adaptogen is a natural, non-habit-forming plant based compound that requires no prescription.

Adaptogens aid in the normalization of your body chemistry. They increase the body's ability to cope with physical stress, emotional stress, stress related imbalances and environmental pollution.

An adaptogen works in a synergistic manner by increasing the body's own ability to fight off illness. Modern drugs on the other hand, tend to target specific disease symptoms after you are sick.

Adaptogens work not only when you take it, but for a sustained period. They become increasingly active the more your body needs it.

These herbs appear to increase the body's ability to adapt to stress and changing situations. They can be taken daily without having to cycle them. These compounds have been used to treat fatigue, stress, and anxiety for thousands of years. They were included in many tonics and drinks before people really understood how they worked. Many European folk remedies contain licorice, a well known adaptogen. In Asia, many people have consumed ginseng for thousands of years as a daily tonic. Native Americans consume their own version of the ginseng species known as American Ginseng.

These unique herbal tonics can lower or raise blood pressure as needed. Adaptogens normalize blood sugar levels helping your immune system gain resistance to diseases. They can also improve overall mental function, increase energy levels, and help you enjoy a good night sleep.

Some of the more common adaptogens can include premier herbs such as Ashwaganda, Siberian Ginseng, Goji Berries, Rhodiola, and Schizandra. Ashwaganda improves weakness or fatigue. Siberian Ginseng has

several benefits worth noting. It can normalize blood pressure, lower cholesterol, regulate blood sugar and strengthen the adrenal glands. Goji can be consumed by eating them raw or soaking them in water until they fill out like grapes. I personally like to eat them daily with my cereal or add them to a healthy shake. According to Chinese herbalists, goji builds the blood and qi in the legs which is great for walkers, runners, martial artist and dancers. This extra circulation of qi in the lower torso is also great for sex.

Goji

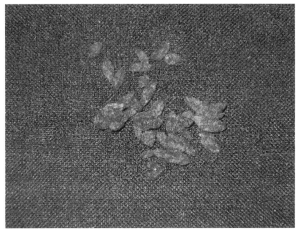

Goji Berries contains polysaccharides that helps to regulate the immune, improve vision and increases libido.

Schizandra Berries

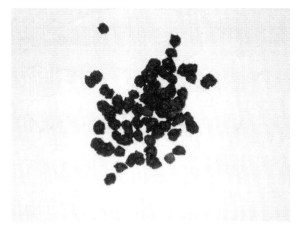

Schizandra Berries improves skin, increases sperm and can prevent premature ejaculation. This herb is said to have all the 5 flavors and an abundance of Qi (energy), Jing (essence) and Shen (spirit) commonly known as the 3 treasures of life.

This herb can increase your energy by stimulating the central nervous system without making you nervous like caffeine. It is considered to be a premier adaptogen. The calming effect of Schizandra helps to mitigate the stressful effects of the hormone cortisol and thereby indirectly protects one's testosterone levels.

Many people take this herb to increase energy. It is especially popular with athletes as it boosts nitric oxide levels in the body. Schizandra is great remedy for fatigue as well. Schizandra increases energy at the cellular level by stimulating the mitrochondria to produce ATP.

The Health Sciences Institute states that Schizandra berries can raise the body's enzyme, glutathione. This enzyme detoxifies the body in a way that improves mental clarity. It is widely taken by students in China for this reason.

Polyrachis or Black Ant (insect viagra)

Black Ant powder is derived from a species of edible black ants common in the Chang Bai Mountains of China and other parts of the world. It is known as the "Herb of Kings" because it was exclusively reserved for the emperors of China as a sexual tonic to help them satisfy their countless concubines. This formulation builds both sexual function and increases virility and fertility. It is anti-aging, good for the immune system and improves the muscle skeletal system. Many athletes and college students in China use black ant daily to keep up with the pace of life.

American Ginseng

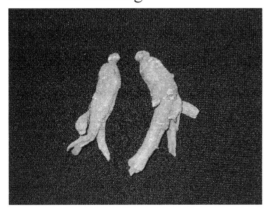

American Ginseng provides a steady supply of energy during the summer months without overheating the body. American Ginseng was used extensively by Native Americans for strength and vitality.

Tibetan Rhodiola is another important herb used by monks in the Tibetan mountains. The monks used this herb to offset the low oxygen levels at high elevations. Tibetan Rhodiola can be useful to treat fatigue, improves overall work performance, reduce symptoms of depression and assist your body to develop a stronger resistance to stress.

How to identify Adaptogens

In order to identify an herb as an adaptogen in nature, three traits must be present. It must be nontoxic to the user in any reasonable amount. The herb must also generate a nonspecific response, meaning that it does not target a specific region of the body but benefits the body as a whole. In addition, the primary function of an adaptogen is to serve and create a state of balance and homeostasis.

In addition to helping the body to adapt to stress, these herbs also appear to be good for people in general. Many of them are high in antioxidants and vitamins. Therefore, before selecting a testosterone booster consider taking an adaptogen herb first to bring the body into balance while protecting it against oxidative stress. Remember stress in general is the number one enemy to any male with regards to sex. Stress can trigger the stress hormone cortisol which in turn can raise insulin levels. As mentioned earlier, insulin can lead to inflammation, lower testosterone levels and increase cell receptor sites for estrogen.

The more extraneous fat a man has, the greater the potential increase in his estrogen level. Estrogen balance is important to men as well when it concerns hormonal balance.

Testosterone and SHBG Chart

Measurements in Conventional Units **(ng/dl)**, SHBG in (nmol/L)							
Age	# Subjects	Total Test.	Stand. Dev.	Free Test.	Stand. Dev.	SHBG	Stand. Dev.
25-34	45	617	170	12.3	2.8	35.5	8.8
35-44	22	668	212	10.3	1.2	40.1	7.9
45-54	23	606	213	9.1	2.2	44.6	8.2
55-64	43	562	195	8.3	2.1	45.5	8.8
65-74	47	524	197	6.9	2.3	48.7	14.2
75-84	48	471	169	6.0	2.3	51.0	22.7
85-100	21	376	134	5.4	2.3	65.9	22.8

Depending upon your age and health, normal total testosterone range for a 20-59-year-old is 270-890 ng/dl. The range for age 60 and above is 352-720 ng/dl.

An ideal T/E ratio is between 40-60:1 for healthy men. Many researchers state that a 50:1 ratio in favor of testosterone to estradiol is just as good. The bad news is that less than 10% achieve these critical ratios and over 75% of them are less than 35 years old. Estrogen in the form of estradiol is useful to men in small amounts and strikes a good balance. When estradiol is in excess it can cause feminine like traits

in men such as male boobs and excess fat around the abdomen. This is called gynecomastia.

The proper selection of herbs or supplements are instrumental when used to increase free testosterone and blood flow to the penis. Every man is different and requires a unique formulation that fits his energy pattern and particular dysfunction. It is important to understand one's constitutional type or strength and weaknesses first. Some men have stronger erections but weaker endurance or staying power. Others have weak erections but no problems with premature ejaculation. Regardless of health problems, all men should have their prostate checked and be disease free.

High blood pressure medication can wreak havoc on blood flow to the penis. Selecting herbs for sex or taking blue pills without understanding one's individual areas of concern can only lead to failure, frustration and a waste of money. Panax Ginseng and Yohimbe may work for some men in combination or may be harmful and impair normal function for others. It all depends upon one's constitutional type and unique metabolic chemistry.

There is a right herb and right women for every man. Take the time and patience to do the proper research and make no assumptions based on popularity, appearances or commercial propaganda. Some men may need to take a kidney yin herb to replenish energy loss as opposed to a kidney yang herb which is used to ignite and express sexual energy. Again, it depends upon a man's make up or constitutional type.

Magnetic Stimulation

Another important adjunct to boosting testosterone often neglected is the judicious use of healing magnets. Magnetic healing has been used for thousand of years by many cultures. I would like to introduce this form of healing to the reader about boosting testosterone and increasing blood flow to the penis. In order to accomplish this task, the south pole polarity is recommended.

South pole energy is used to stimulate organ function, increase hormones and strengthen weaknesses when there is no pain, tumor or infection present. The south pole end of the magnet should not be used if you are ill, have pain or an active infection.

In order to increase testosterone, place the south end pole of the magnet just below the testicles while in a lying or sitting position or sandwich the magnet

between the penis and testicles for about 15-20 minutes daily. Assess your progress weekly.

The strength of magnet is measured in gauss. A strong magnet can range in gauss from usually 1,000 – 3500 gauss. If you have a 500- gauss magnet its power can be amplified by combining 3 magnets back to back to increase its output to 1500 gauss (3 X 500 gauss). Placing the south pole magnet on the adrenal glands can also increase their function.

One more useful tip using magnets entails placing a glass of water on top of the south pole end of a magnet for about 30 minutes and drinking it at room temperature. Drinking south pole magnetic water can energize your system thus providing more yang power for sex. For more detail explanation on the proper use of magnets see reference sources on the next page.

Sexual Intercourse

Having sex 2 or more times a week can certainly wake up one's sleeping giant and testosterone. The rise in T levels are usually the result of the supply and demand placed upon the testicles. Men should however be advised that excessive ejaculation can render a man dry of passion and zeal. Don't forget to practice edging.

Sexual Positions

The ancient text of the Karma Sutra written thousands of years ago in India, teaches us that some positions are better than others for certain individuals. The careful selection of these erotic postures can impact sexual performance in a positive way. Based upon my own research and anecdotal testimonies of others, I have concluded that there are 3 primary sexual positions every man should master.

Missionary Position (MP)

Benefits: This position describes the classic romantic way of having sex with the man lying on top of the woman. MP is good for those men who are prone to premature ejaculation due to over excitement. This position helps a man learn self control, breathing and seminal retention. It is yin in nature.

The missionary position can foster lots of harmony, balance and
bonding between a couple. The missionary position is a great position to finish out a night of passionate love making.

Dog Position: (DP)

Benefits: This position describes a woman being on her knees while the man enters her from the rear. The DP is great for arousal in those men who have low libido and weak erections. This position is very yang in nature and should be practiced with moderation or by men who have lots of control. DP can easily cause the average man to lose control prematurely while failing to satisfy his mate.

Riding the Surf Position (RSP)

Benefits:

In this position, a woman straddles a man while he is lying down. This position helps to preserves a man's yang energy and really excites a woman to have multiple orgasms. It is a great position to use for women who are difficult to satisfy, have a high sex drive or require lots of stimulation. The RSP gives women a sense that they are in control of their own orgasm, which excites them even further.

References:

1. Magnetic Healing, by Buryl Payne, Ph.D copyright 1995

2. Biomagnetic and Herbal Therapy, by Michael Tierra, copyright 1997

3. Radiant Health on Chinese Tonic Herbs, by Ron Teeguarden, copyright 1998

Adaptogens:

http://www.ehow.com/about_5427002_adaptogens.html#ixzz2wbCVrMyK

http://www.ehow.com/about_5427002_adaptogens.html#ixzz2wbCjTGPz

Chapter 13

STACKING, FEEDBACK LOOP AND CYCLING

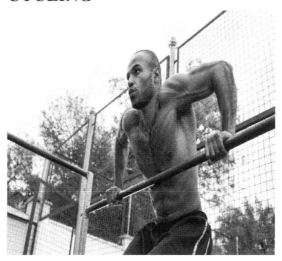

After having made the right selection each man needs to consider the concept of stacking. What is stacking? Stacking is an approach that emphasizes the use of a group of supplements to enhance performance rather than reliance upon one. Herbs and supplements tend to be more powerful in their effect when used in synergistic harmony and properly combined.

A combination of supplements can be more effective than those taken individually. If properly integrated in a formula, the results can prove to be quite rewarding. Stacking also feature products with different intended purposes that work together to enhance energy, endurance and recovery.

Stacking supplements essentially means putting two or more products together to help enhance results. Certain supplements feed off of one another. A good example of stacking would be a mix of Tribulus Terrestris, ZMA and L-arginine. Tribulus in itself has been shown to raise natural testosterone by 30%, stacked along side with ZMA which also aids in natural testosterone production. MA is a natural mineral supplement made up of zinc, magnesium aspartate, and vitamin B6. Zinc supports your immune system and muscles. Magnesium plays a role in metabolism and muscle health and helps manage sleep. The addition of B6 may boost energy.

In 2000, researchers gave ZMA supplement to a group of NCAA football players working out twice a day. After 7 weeks, they found a significant increase in the players' testosterone and growth, both of which are linked to muscle growth. However, one of the scientists who conducted the study holds the registered trademark for the original formula of ZMA, and his company funded the research. This combination will help to build lean muscle mass, increase energy levels, and improve erections.

L-arginine helps target blood flow to the penis. Lack of blood flow is usually a major cause of erectile dysfunction. One of the best stacking programs that I would recommend is the combination of HGH and testosterone.

What is a HGH/Testosterone Stack?

Dr. Mercola, a well-known proponent of health and wellness advocates in his newsletters the judicious use of both HGH and testosterone precursor booster. He proposes that complete rejuvenation can better be achieved when you replenish your HGH and testosterone levels at the same time. This is called a HGH testosterone stack. The HGH testosterone stack has a compound effect far greater than either of the

two hormones used individually. Dr. Mercola suggests that testosterone helps our human growth hormones to work faster thus increasing cell efficiency and recovery from a workout.

Natural HGH encourages the pituitary gland to generate more of the particular pure HGH. As soon as it is discharged directly into the system, the natural HGH starts revitalizing various systems of the body.

Areas of concentration are the testicles of which increase the generation of testosterone. It is the testosterone that improves muscle production and more importantly sexual desire.

The HGH/testosterone stack method can greatly assist in fat loss as well as muscle building. The HGH/testosterone stack has been shown to restore focus, energy, sex drive and performance to more youthful levels.

Our next topic is about understanding the Negative Feedback Loop (NFL) concept. This term defines a situation in which the more you do something for a positive gain, the greater chance for a loss. Wikipedia defines the (NFL) as occurring when the result of a process influences the operation of the process itself in such a way as to reduce changes. When synthetic testosterone is used repeatedly our brain begins to send message to the body to shut down its own natural production. This is ot good and should be avoided at all cost. The best approach would be to increase a man's natural production using precursors of testosterone thus avoiding the use of anabolic synthetic hormones altogether.

This approach leads us to the principle called cycling.

What is Cycling?

Cycling is based upon a ratio of using a particular product for a specific period of time and then discontinuing usage until a certain time interval has expired. The obvious purpose of cycling is to avoid building tolerance to a supplement. Once tolerance is reached a higher dosage will be necessary to achieve the same effect, unless one cycles. A typical cycle ratio is usually 2: 1 or I day off for every 2 days on. I personally have achieved good results with a 5 day on 2 days off schedule.

A good example of cycling can be demonstrated by taking a supplement such as Tongkat Ali for a duration of 7 days on and 4 days off to avoid tolerance.

Daily Rotation of supplements can be considered an upgraded form of cycling that promises even better results than straight cycling. Here's how it works. Take one capsule of a product the first day. The next day take one capsule of another product, and

repeat for 7 days. This program is great if you are well organized and dedicated. You will need seven different testosterone boosters or 7 bottles. At the end of the week take a few days off and resume.

Consult with your doctor if you have health issues or taking medications. Many sexual performance programs rarely mention any of these principles and are doomed to fail or have only a short window of success. They may work for a week or even less. Most of the erections achieved are usually short lived.

How does an erection work?

The proper sequential pattern of achieving a firm erection can be illustrated by the following conversions:

Citrulline > Arginine > Nitric Oxide > Guanylate Cyclase > Relaxation of the Corpora Cavernosa = "Penile Erection"

Intrinsic Areas of Concern to be Addressed.

Here are some of the problem areas that all men need to monitor in addressing sexual fitness and libido.

Conversion of Testosterone to Estrogen (estradiol)
Estrogen can cause prostate swelling.
Sex Hormone Binding Globulin SHBG can neutralize healthy testosterone before it is delivered to the target area.
Low levels Nitric Oxide (NO) Blood does not flow well when the arteries are not wide open.

5 Alpha Reductase is the enzyme that triggers the conversion of testosterone to DHT, this is only a problem if DHT is in excess in the body.

Adequate amounts of DHT are beneficial to men and is more powerful androgenic effect than testosterone itself.

PDE5 or Phosphodiesterase type 5 activates an enzyme that causes erectile dysfunction.

Aromatase is an enzyme that contributes to the conversion of testosterone to estrogen.

Guanosine Monophosphate or cGMP dysfunction can cause a reduction in the blood flow to the penis. Enhancing GMP levels can increase contractions of the heart muscle, help the arteries and other smooth muscles to relax, increases the secretion of insulin and lipolysis (fat destruction). Best of all, GMP makes your workouts easier, and erections harder while burning fat.

Xenoestrogens from the environment can cause excess estrogen in the blood.

Stress both acute and chronic can result in adrenal burnout and high cortisol levels.

Low Free Flowing Testosterone this is the bioactive form that circulates in the blood stream causing a man to feel manly and sexual.

<u>Performance Anxiety</u>. When you feel that your best is not good enough due to unrealistic expectation such as being a super stud or porn star.

<u>Sexual Hormone Binding Globulin ("SHBG")</u>

This hormone captures and neutralizes free testosterone ("FT"). In order to maximize the amount of testosterone, the hijacker aromatase (converts T to estrogen) must be controlled in addition to managing 5-alpha-reductase.

I recommend that all sexual warriors seriously consider the consumption of the following nutrients to protect themselves from testosterone ambush:

SHBG: use Tonkat Ali to fight SHBG
Aromatase: Block aromatase by using resveratrol, genistein, chrysin, quercetin, beta-sitosterol
5-alpha-reductase inhibitors.

The new age sexual warrior should always strive to maximize T levels and DHT and minimize (E) estrogen. The All of these important areas of concern can negatively impact a man's sexual performance. Once these problem areas are assessed and addressed properly, a sexual warrior will then begin to see a dramatic improvement in the bedroom.

It is also imperative that every man should have a tailored program of supplementation that will target their own areas of concern. For some men, there may be more areas of concerns in contrast to others. For example, one man may have problems with excess DHT, aromatase and PDE5, while another may suffer from exposure to xenoestrogens and low levels of nitric oxide. Once again, I emphasize the fact that one shoe does not fit all and the need for a more diversified approach.

Benign Prostatic Hyperplasia (BPH) or enlarged prostate is the number one medical diagnosis for men over 55 in America. Eighty percent of American men will experience some problems associated with their prostates. In order to keep your prostate gland functioning normally and within the range of a healthy-size, I would suggest taking the following supplements.

* Bee Pollen - 1000mg, 2 times per day

* Boron - 3 to 6mg, once per day

* Stinging Nettle Root - 300mg, once a day. Make sure this is nettle "root" not nettle "leaf"

Pumpkin Seed Extract - 200mg, 2 times per day

Saw Palmetto Root – 400mg twice daily

Pygeum Africanum – 25mg 2 times daily

During the cycling phase of taking supplements one should take into account, PCT or post cycling therapy. This period represents a time when one has cycled off of all supplements but need to maintain the gains made with them. One of the much talked about breakthroughs in research for men is a supplement known as D-aspartic acid or DAA. It is now available to help resolve the down time between cycling.

Anabolic Steroids

When we supplement with anabolic androgenic steroids or PED ,performance enhancement drugs , our natural hormone levels are altered. Most anabolic steroids tend to suppress our natural testosterone production to one degree or another. If we're not careful our estrogen and progesterone levels can increase beyond a healthy range resulting in hypogonadism or shrinking of the testicles. Estrogen and progesterone can both be controlled while on cycle with proper supplementation practices. Steroids can cause testosterone suppression to will remain for several years.

When we discontinue steroid use, testosterone levels are still in a suppressed state.

It's often recommended you stimulate natural production and let your body normalize. While testosterone stimulation is the primary purpose, the normalization factor of a post cycle therapy plan is of great importance. DAA can increase testosterone levels as much as 42% over the course of a 12 day off cycle by stimulating the release of luteinizing hormones from the pituitary gland.

How does D-aspartic acid work?

D-aspartic acid increases natural testosterone production by increasing the release of gonadotrophin and luteinizing hormones. DAA triggers the release of the GnRH (gonadotropin) hormone that informs the pituitary that testosterone concentration in the blood is falling. Oxytocin and vasopressin (the love hormones), luteinizing hormone (LH) and the growth hormone (GH) are also released from the pituitary gland. The pituitary gland and the testes have the ability to trap circulating D-aspartic acid.

Natural increased release of GnRH and LH resulting in increased testosterone levels can be observed from puberty only to mid-twenties.

Men after 30 experience lowered testosterone levels leading to a lowered libido, increased body fat levels, problems with sleep, decreased recovery ability, and decreased ability to build up muscle. Here's the bottom line, DAA supplement causes your body to produce more testosterone as if you were younger and helps to get rid of the above-mentioned symptoms.

The deciding advantage of D-aspartic acid over direct testosterone supplementation (e.g. with steroids) is that it allows for testosterone to be produced by your body and not delivered from outside. Synthetic testosterone poses an imbalance by interfering with the body's own testosterone production. Increased testosterone levels triggered by DAA benefits sexual performance and muscle growth.

The sex hormone testosterone enhances libido and erection quality, intensifies perceived orgasm and extends duration of intercourse. Testosterone makes your energy level rise in contrast to low T which is responsible for depression and lowered life satisfaction. By elevating testosterone level,

D- aspartic acid makes your workouts more effective and helps you build muscle. Stimulation with DAA acid increases cyclic adenosine monophosphate (AMP) in the receiving nerves. AMP is a cell-regulating compound, probably the most important one. It plays an important role in the cellular reaction on hormones.

D-Aspartic acid has been suggested to help promote normal GABA levels while dopamine levels function as an anti-depressant. Another benefit of

DAA is its ability to increase nitric oxide (NO2, NO3) production and its blood level, promoting fast recovery after workouts. D-aspartic acid is one of the newest natural testosterone boosters available on the market.

You can buy DAA supplements in the form of pure DAA or stacked with other testosterone boosters, which is convenient. It is always a good idea to stack DAA with other testosterone boosters that don't already contain DAA. Pure DAA is available in form of DAA powder and is manufactured here in the USA. The DAA dosage used in many research studies recommend 3 grams taken in the morning.

The manufactures of the DAA supplement suggests a loading phase of five days, with 3 grams applied in the morning and another 3 grams in the evening.

What about side effects of DAA?

The journal "Impulse" reported that D-aspartic acid can cause seizures and increase the likelihood of alzheimer's disease due to **excess activation of aspartate receptors**. Risk for other nervous system disorders such as amyotrophic lateral sclerosis and Hungtington's disease is elevated as well. Keep in mind the term excess activation. Like any other substance use it as intended and avoid misuse or overuse.

As with all testosterone boosters, I would suggest you cycle it as well to avoid building up a tolerance or excess activation of aspartate receptors.

This is easy to do when you use it between cycles of other supplements. In fact, another manufacturer of the DAA supplement suggested a cycle 2 weeks on and 1 week off. Discover and experiment what works best for you.

References:

D'Aniello A. D-Aspartic acid: an endogenous amino acid with an important neuroendocrine role. Brain Res Rev. 2007 Feb;53(2):215-34.

Pinilla L, Tena-Sempere M, Aguilar E. Role of excitatory amino acid pathways in control of gonadotrophin secretion in adult female rats sterilized by neonatal administration of oestradiol or testosterone. J Reprod Fertil. 1998 May;113(1):53-9.

Topo E, Soricelli A, D'Aniello A, Ronsini S, D'Aniello G. The role and molecular mechanism of D-aspartic acid in the release and synthesis of LH and testosterone in humans and rats. Reprod Biol Endocrinol. 2009 Oct 27;7:120.

D'Aniello A, Di Fiore MM, D'Aniello G, Colin FE, Lewis G, Setchell BP. Secretion of D-aspartic acid by the rat testis and its role in endocrinology of the testis and spermatogenesis. FEBS Lett. 1998 Sep 25;436(1):23-7.

D'Aniello A, Di Cosmo A, Di Cristo C, Annunziato L, Petrucelli L, Fisher G. Involvement of D-aspartic acid in the synthesis of testosterone in rat testes. Life Sci. 1996;59(2):97-104.

Nagata Y, Homma H, Matsumoto M, Imai K. Stimulation of steroidogenic acute regulatory protein (StAR) gene expression by D-aspartate in rat Leydig cells. FEBS Lett. 1999 Jul 9;454(3):317-20.

Chapter 14

FIRST AID SEX HERBS

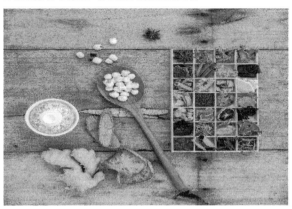

We will now review in more detail how supplementation with herbs can help to address specific key problem areas that can inhibit sexual functioning. First on our list is a herb known as stinging nettle.

Stinging Nettle has numerous benefits, including unbinding testosterone, inhibiting the production of excess DHT which can negatively impacts male health). It also helps to neutralize the sex-hormone binding globulin (SHBG). The good news is that, nettle root can increase free testosterone and maintain DHT at healthy levels, making both readily available for use.

Nettle root helps block the conversion of testosterone into estrogen and relieve prostate issues.

Nettle root has been shown to decrease night time urination frequency, improve urination power, and help shrink enlarged prostate tissue.

Make sure you take the root extract form of nettle instead of the nettle leaf. Lucky for us all, nettle root is inexpensive and widely available.

Why is Saw Palmetto good for you?

Saw Palmetto inhibits the enzyme 5 alpha reductase that converts testosterone into DHT. Keep in mind that more than often DHT is not the problem while estrogen is in prostate tissue. Saw Palmetto is the specific herb in many herbal formulas that's used to improve male potency, reproductive problems, the reduction of inflammation and swelling of the prostate gland. It provides the necessary nutrition and strengthens all glands in the body. Saw Palmetto is the best-known for its affect on sexual function.

It has a strong affinity for the reproductive and nervous systems. When the prostate enlarges, testosterone levels build up in the prostate gland causing the formation of estrogen. It is estrogen not DHT that cause the prostate cells to multiply at an accelerated rate. The fat-soluble saw palmetto berries prevent this chemical conversion which blocks the rapid abnormal cell growth of the prostate gland or BPH process. Another rogue enzyme responsible for erectile dysfunction is caused by PDE-5 working against the enzyme cGMP. cGMP is one of the enzymes that help your body to make nitric oxide. PDE inhibitors like Viagra, Levitra and Cialis work by deactivating PDE-5 which in turn increases cGMP to produce more nitric oxide.

Most males turn immediately to PDE inhibitors such as, Viagra, without even considering a less expensive safer alternative. Herbal alternatives have been used by men effectively for decades and even centuries without negative side effects. PDE-5 inhibitors such as Cialis and Levitra are not without side effects and are highly questionable for long term use.

Many men have already experienced the benefits of taking herbs while noticing results within a matter of a week or two in some cases. Furthermore, many herbal compounds have a positive dualistic positive effect by increasing both libido and testosterone.

Another good example of what is available and safe to take for men of all ages for erectile dysfunction issues and libido is an amino acid called L-Citrulline.

Citrulline is the new wonder supplement on the block. A natural food source of citrulline is the red and yellow watermelon. Most of the citrulline is found in the rind of the watermelon.

The yellow watermelon contains 4 times as much citrulline as the more popular red version. One would need to eat about 1.5 lb. of the red watermelon to receive a therapeutic dosage of Citrulline. Sixty percent of the watermelon rind contains most of the citrulline needed to trigger the body's release of l-arginine.

The beauty of Citrulline is that even small amounts will increase baseline nitric oxide levels, especially in men with endothelial dysfunction. A Citrulline supplement can be combined with arginine for a more synergistic potency and longer period of enhanced blood flow. A minimum dosage of 200 mg – ,000 mg combined with 4 -6 grams of Arginine is needed to duplicate the nitric oxide release of Cialis for a 24-36-hour window of readiness. This is absolutely critical, because most middle-aged and beyond men with erection-related issues are in this category. Viagra and Cialis will often not work for older men because they simply do not have enough nitric oxide in their arteries for these medications to act upon.

Korean ginseng sometimes referred to as
Panax Ginseng has been one of the big guns in erectile research and has a fairly established track record. In fact, it has been used literally for centuries. Its potent sexual powers come from its ability to directly boost nitric oxide, a fact that has been verified in multiple

animal and human studies. Furthermore, several studies have showed that it actually helps with erectile dysfunction.

Icariin Extract.
 Icariin, chief phyto-chemical in Wild Horny Goat Weed, gives this herb its erectile superpowers. Viagra and Cialis are PDE-5 inhibitors and icariin is one as well. It is significantly less powerful than Viagra and Cialis. Make sure you opt for the 10% or higher potency extracts to increase its effectiveness.
Icariin also has antioxidant and other properties that seem to give it actual healing properties. Many men have had excellent results with products such as wild goat horny weed at a dosage of 1,000mg containing 10% Icariin.

CoQ10, known as coenzyme Q10 has many excellent properties and has been extensively studied. It is well-known for its mitochondrial protective powers and is used in alternative medicine for a variety of conditions, including gum disease. But what few men know is that it also helps the body preserve nitric oxide levels. It has been shown in several studies to increase blood flow. The benefits are mostly for those men 40 or older and those with endothelial dysfunction. The best form of this supplement is ubiquinol which is 10 times more potent than regular CoQ10.

Fish Oil is not directly an erectile supplement, but I mention it here because of one European study found that it helped endothelial function and nitric oxide output in diabetic patients. Yet another study found that fish oil helps to increase the elasticity of arteries. As males, we always want nice expandable blood vessels that allow blood to flow into the penis. Fish oil is also known to protect against inflammation and triglycerides which can clog up penile arteries. It may even optimize free testosterone while doing its thing. Fish oil benefits both the heart and penis.
CAUTION! It's very easy to buy rancid fish oil, which will do more

harm than good. Make sure your fish oil is not contaminated with mercury and PCB's. Shop wisely! A really good bran to consider is Nordic

Gingko

Gingko, like Pycnogenol, strengthens the activity of nitric oxide synthesis (NOS), making it a viable erectile dysfunction supplement. Furthermore, animal studies have shown that gingko relaxes dependent arteries including those all-important ones supplying blood to the penis. Direct evidence that gingko improves erectile dysfunction and impotence is still lacking in some arenas of research. Any herb that can increase nitric oxide levels in men is an asset. Gingko is one of these herbs and can be purchased inexpensively. Gingko has shown promise in improving erections in men with erectile dysfunction that resulted from taking antidepressants.

CAUTION! Care should be exercised with supplements such as gingko because they tend to thin the blood and may interfere with drug interactions such as NSAIDS and anticoagulants.

Deer Antler

The Chinese and Russians both stake high claims on the benefits of deer antler. It is known to balance the endocrine system, including curing or enhancing the treatment of penile erectile dysfunction in men.

Deer Antler is beneficial for men with watery semen, enlarged prostate glands and impotence.

Deer Antler acts as both a male and female sex hormone, freeing up and circulating more testosterone in the blood system. It is a natural and effective aphrodisiac. As a natural inflammatory agent many athletes use it for speedy recovery from workouts.

Tribulus Terretris

Now we will investigate in more detail another one of the superstars of aphrodisiacs previously mentioned, tribulus. Tribulus seems to work quite well by increasing DHEA, libido and nitric oxide. Tribulus (sometimes called – puncture vine, devil's weed has been marketed for ages as a natural testosterone / libido booster.

Tribulus contains some very interesting steroidal like substances called saponins. One of which is called protodioscin. A minimum standardized extract of 45% or higher saponins of protodiocin is highly recommended to enhance results. Protodioscin is a chemical "cousin" of DHEA, a steroid hormone produced by the adrenal glands. It is the only "hormone" not affected by the U.S. prohormone ban of 2005.

On the sexual side of things, Tribulus does appear to be a relatively reliable and potent libido enhancer in rats and humans. Many studies have confirmed an increase in sexual well being and erectile function. While it is not exactly known how Tribulus works, it is known to enhance androgen receptor density in the brain (muscle tissue not confirmed) which may enhance the libido enhancing properties of androgens.

Limited evidence suggests that it is weak to non-effective in enhancing fertility. Tribulus is a plant that has been used for generations in ayurvedic medicine. The root and fruits are used for male virility and general vitality. The root tendS to enhance libido and sexual well being without affecting testosterone while the fruit appear to be potently protective of organ function. In cases for individuals who are trying to avoid increased testosterone due to medical reasons, may find Tribulus to be a safer alternative for enhancing libido. It is always prudent to check with your physician before taking Tribulus to rule out any unwarranted side effects.

How should Tribulus be taken?

Based on a 60% saponin extract, a dose of between 200-450 mg a day is typically used for libido enhancement and sexuality. A concentrated extract dosage of 1,000 mg is highly recommended with a minimun saponin content of 45% or higher.

If rodent research applies to humans, then the dosage of 5mg/kg of Tribulus saponins which is seen as the optimal dose would correlate to a human dosage of:

55 mg saponins (90 mg of a 60% extract)

70 mg saponins (120 mg of a 60% extract)

90 mg saponins (150 mg of a 60% extract)

It would seem that low doses are better. If a concentrated extract is not used, traditional dosages of the basic root powder are in the 5-6-gram range.

Ok, it time to deal with the big boy on the block, who goes by the name Tongkat Ali also known as Asian or Malaysia Viagra. It is considered to be one of the most effective non-prescriptive herbs for naturally increasing testosterone in both men and women without dangerous side effects. Tongkat is grown in the rainforest of Malaysia and Indonesia.

It is a form of ginseng. Tongkat Ali is a very well known southeast Asian herbal remedy that is also called Eurycoma Longifolia or simply Longjack. The root is the most potent part of the tree. The key compounds must be extracted in a special way. Simply grinding up the root into a powder is not effective or advisable. Special extraction methods must be employed.

This herb is more effective than Tribulus in producing luteinizing hormones. These are hormones if you recall that stimulate the testicles to produce more testosterone without side effects. Tongkat can increase energy, stamina, athletic ability and libido in men and women as well without side effects. Based upon the study of the The British Journal of Sports Medicine, Tongkat Ali indeed appears to be a strong testosterone booster. Taking Tongkat Ali can cause sexual performance to be boosted in a variety of ways:

-More intense orgasms
-Dramatic boost in libido
-Increases semen volume
* increases testosterone

* decreases male menopausal issues
* increases energy levels
* improves overall mood
* improves erectile function and frequency
* promotes muscle growth and recovery after workouts
* may increase sperm count and mobility thereby increasing fertility

It's best to cycle Tongkat Ai so you don't build up a tolerance over time. My recommendation is 5 days on at the max, then at least 2 days off before starting up again. Mix it up with other T boosters to keep your body guessing!

There are of course many other great aphrodisiacs many too numerous to mention in this book in detail. I have only highlighted those T boosters that are more popular and accessible to almost anyone for a reasonable price.

 If you are on medication, work with your doctor to get off of the medications whenever possible. If your doctor is not willing to help you get off your medications or synthetic hormones, fire him and find someone who will. There are doctors out there who won't attempt to medicate or over medicate patients the minute they walk through the front door.

Keep in mind that testosterone boosters were never Intended to be a total panacea. These supplements should be used as part of a comprehensive holistic lifestyle to enhance everything else you're doing. Testosterone boosters are great to have and take on a rotational basis provided that nitric oxide levels are optimal and balanced.

References:

Phytotherapy Research 2002,16:1-5; Nutrition Research,2001,21:1251-1260;Nutrition Research, 2003,23: 1189-1198;Life Sciences,2004,74:855-862

2) J Urol 2002; 168:2070-3

3) Asian J Androl 2007;9(2):241-4

4) Intl Journ Cardio 2005 Feb 28, 98(3):413-9

5) Eur Heart Journ 2007 28(18):2249-2255

6) Urology 2004 Apr,63(4):641-646

7) Curr Med Res Opin, 2004 Sep,20(9):1377-1384

8) Amer Jour Clin Nutr, 2007 Sep,86(3):610-7

9) Amer Jour Cardio,2007 Aug 1,100(3):455-8

10) Am Jour Clin Nutr, Apr 2007, 85(4):1068-74

11) J Cardiovasc Pharmacol,1998,32:509-515

12) Hum Psychopharmacol,2002,17:279-284

13) Gen Pharmacol,1982,13:169-171;Gen Pharmacol,1982,13:225-230;Gen Pharmacol,1983,14:277-280

14) J Clin 17) Gen Pharmacol,1982,13:169-171;Gen Pharmacol,1982,13:225-230;Gen Pharmacol,1983,14:277-280

15) J Clin Endocrinol Metab,1991,73:4-7

16) Eur J Clin Nutr, 2008 Dec, 62(12):1426-31, Epub 2007, "Fish oil supplementation improves large

arterial elasticity in overweight hypertensive patients",
Wang, et. al.

17) Journal of Andrology, Sep/Oct 2008,(29):5

18) JAMA,2007,297:2351-2359932-40
19) Circulation, 1998 Jun 9, 97(22):2222-9
20) Intl J Impotence Res, 2008, 20:173-180
21)) Intl J Impotence Res, 2008, 20:173-180
22) Eur J Clin Nutr, 2008 Dec, 62(12):1426-31, Epub
2007, "Fish oil supplementa26) Eur J Clin Nutr, 2008
Dec, 62(12):1426-31, Epub 2007, "Fish oil
supplementation improves large arterial elasticity in
overweight hypertensive patients", Wang, et. al.
23) Journal of Chromatography A, 17 June 2005,
1078(1-2):196-200, "Determination of citrulline in
watermelon rind"
24) Brit J Sports Med, Oct 2003, 37: 464–70. "The
Ergogenic Effects of Eurycoma Longifolia Jack: A
Pilot Study"
25) Article Source: http://EzineArticles.com/2267596
. This herb is extracted from the roots of the Pasak
Bumi tree.
Read more at:
http://www.ehow.com/facts_5008655_what-benefits-
tongkat-ali.html#ixzz2yEuee4tK

http://EzineArticles.com/2267596

Chapter 15

Nitric Oxide
The High Performance Compound

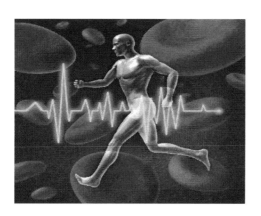

Nitric oxide (N-O) is crucial for optimum health. It helps to relax the arteries, thus regulating healthy blood pressure and increasing circulation and oxygen delivery to every system, organ, and tissue in the body. N-O helps to regulate blood flow to the cells and ensure nutrient absorption. It also provides immune support.

Nitric oxide is a gas molecule that is released within endothelial cells and plays a critical role in several functions in the body, including reducing inflammation, kidney function and oxygen transport. In addition, nitric oxide helps relax and dilate blood vessels, which increases blood flow in the body. This can have positive effects on blood pressure as well as heart health. Evidence indicates that changing your dietary and exercise program can increase nitric oxide levels in the body. Consult your health-care provider before taking any supplements.

As we age, our body produces less nitric oxide which renders our blood flow less than optimal.

The side effect of poor blood flow is quite apparent to those over the age of 40. Older men tend to struggle with wound healing, hair loss, fatigue, certain types of memory loss and erectile dysfunction or ED.

During the course of my research, I discovered that beet root contains a high concentration of dietary nitrates. Well you probably thought nitrites are bad for you. Nitrites are often used as an additive to hot dogs and meats are known carcinogens when tested on lab rats. This form of nitrite is bad and should be avoided. Like cholesterol you have the good and the bad form in the body. The nitrates in beets are converted to a healthy form of nitrites in the body.

Feel free to indulge yourself when it comes to beets. When consumed in sufficient quantities beets can significantly increase nitric oxide in the body. Nitric oxide is responsible for decreases in blood pressure by signaling the blood vessels to expand allowing more blood flow. More blood flow means harder erection.

Benefits of Nitric Oxide

Maintain healthy blood pressure

Support normal triglyceride levels

Enhance healthy circulation

Promote artery health

Support cardiovascular and heart health

Improve exercise endurance and performance

Support sexual performance via improved circulations

How Nitric Oxide Works

Nitric oxide is produced by three main enzymes called nitric oxide synthase (NOS). The NOS that has to do with erectile dysfunction is found in the endothelial cells of blood vessels in the penis. This enzyme breaks down l-arginine to create N-O, nitric oxide, which stimulates the cells to produce cyclic GMP or guanosine monophosphate. GMP regulates the movement of ions while signaling the smooth muscle in the blood vessels to relax. Phosphodiesterases, or PDE (sometimes called PDE-5), degrade the GMP, which causes the blood vessels to constrict. PDE-5 is most concentrated in the lungs and penis. There are numerous other substances on the market that can address erectile dysfunction besides drugs.

Nitric oxide supplements can come in a variety of natural forms that affect the same systems. One of them is horny goat weed (the name says it all) which contains a chemical called icariin in it. Icariin has been found to act as a PDE-5 inhibitor which can enhance the production of nitric oxide, it also mimics testosterone. Wild Goat Horny Weed is also known as Epimedium.

Wild Goat Horny Weed or Epimedium, is also called randy cow grass. Remember that, without nitric oxide there is no sex! Nitric Oxide levels must always be of primary concern for the sexual warrior and monitored properly.

A common mistake many men make is in thinking that their testosterone levels are low before first checking out the level of nitric oxide (N0) in the blood. Men need to boost their nitric oxide naturally while increasing testosterone levels. Proven nitric oxide boosters like l-arginine, l-citrulline, arginine and alpha-ketoglutarate, or **AAKG**, (a combination of the amino acid Arginine with an Alpha-ketogluterate molecule) will have a more immediate effect.

Testosterone can have dramatic effect on a man's health when combined with nitric oxide.

Higher testosterone levels make you strong, quick, smart, and aggressive. On workout days, take L-Arginine 30 minutes before your workout. On off days, take it before bed on an empty stomach. Only take the natural "L" form of this amino acid. Studies show that taking Citrulline can result in higher arginine levels in your blood than by taking arginine alone. When combined you get a greater synergistic impact.

Other tips for increasing one's production of nitric oxide are plentiful. Let's start with exercises. Ok, What's the deal? The deal is daily exercises.

Exercise Daily
When you exercise, whether it be running or lifting weights, your body needs more oxygen. Exercise causes the heart to pump harder due to the increase of arterial pressure resulting in more nitric oxide. The increase of nitric oxide widens the arteries and thus allows for more oxygen and blood to circulate.

Supplement with l-arginine and l-citrulline whenever possible. These two amino acids improve nitric oxide levels, according to a study conducted by lead author

Edzard Schwedhelm and colleagues from the University Medical Centre Hamburg-Eppendorf in Germany. The report, which was published in the January 2008 issue of the "British Journal of Clinical Pharmacology," revealed that subjects taking 3 grams each of l-arginine and l-citrulline per day for one week experienced increases in nitric oxide levels compared to those taking a placebo.

These amino acids are generally safe taken at this dosage, but might cause digestive upset in some people.

Eating foods high in antioxidants like garlic and blueberries can protect the nitric oxide your body produces by fighting off free radicals which can damage it. We can protect those enzymes and nitric oxide by consuming healthy foods and antioxidants, like fruit, garlic, vitamins C and E, Co-Q10, and alpha lipoic acid, allowing you to produce more nitric oxide. The more antioxidant protection we provide, the more stable nitric oxide levels will be and the longer it will last.

Nutritious Beets

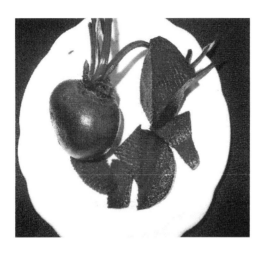

We will now go deeper into the subject of why beets are healthy for us. Once again, we all need to beef up the beets. Beets have long been associated with blood. After all, it is red and loaded with iron and compounds that can dramatically boost nitric oxide in the blood as stated previously. Organic raw beet root provides a wide range of nutrients. Its most significant phytochemical is betaine. This plant chemical helps the liver and kidneys recycle the amino acid methionine to maintain the body's stores of S-adenosyl-methionine, more commonly known as SAM-e. Betaine also helps the liver process fat preventing the accumulation of fatty tissues in the liver (steatosis), especially in heavy drinkers. It also helps moderate triglycerides and LDL cholesterol in the blood. The American Heart Association recommends beet juice to promote healthy blood pressure.

Organic beet root is a wonderful cleansing and nourishing tonic that builds the blood, particularly improving the blood quality for menstruating women.

Beets normalize the blood's pH balance (reducing acidity) and purifies the blood by flushing away fatty deposits and improving circulation. Further supporting its role as a blood purifier, beet root has been used to detoxify and heal the liver and spleen.

Beets are high in many vitamins and minerals such as potassium, magnesium, fiber, phosphorus, iron, vitamins A, B & C; beta-carotene, beta-cyanine and folic acid. These are but a few of the many nutrients, vitamins and minerals that can be found in beets and beet greens. Beets are "Nature's Viagra Vegetable."

One of the first known uses of beets was documented by the ancient Romans, who used them medicinally as an aphrodisiac. Beets are not just an urban legend. Science backs it up too. Beets contain high amounts of boron, which is directly related to the production of human sex hormones.

As I said before, beets are high in natural nitrates, which are converted to nitric oxide in the body. Nitric oxide is known to expand the walls of blood vessels so you can enjoy more oxygen, more nutrients, and more energy. Studies have shown nitric oxide to increase the efficiency of the mitochondria (your energy powerhouses). The results of some research studies demonstrate that a single small serving (70 ml) of beetroot juice can reduced resting blood pressure by as much as 2%.

A single small serving also increased the length of time professional divers could hold their breath by 11%. Cyclists who drank a single larger serving (500 ml) of beetroot juice were able to ride up to 20% longer. Beets can increase blood flow due to their nitrates. Increased blood flow to the genital areas is one of the mechanisms Viagra and other pharmaceuticals use to create this effect. Beets can also be used to test ph level of the stomach. If you are eating a lot of beets or drinking beet juice, and your urine turns pink, guess what? You probably have low stomach acid. Nutritionists can now make good use of beets and beet juice to test stomach acid levels in a safe non-invasive way.

References:

1. Shinde UA, Mehta AA, Goyal RK. Nitric Oxide: a molecule of the millennium. Indian J Exp Biol 2000 Mar;38(3):201-10.

2. Furchgott RF, Ignarro LJ, Murad F. Discover concerning nitric oxide as a signaling molecule in the cardiovascular system. Nobel Prize in Medicine and Physiology 1998.

3. Guoyao W, Meininger CJ. Arginine Nutrition and Cardiovascular Function. J Nutr.2000;130: 2626-2629

4. Seidler M, Uckert S, Waldkirch E, Stief CG, Oelke M, Tsikas D, Sohn M, Jonas U. In vitro effects of a novel class of nitric oxide (NO) donating compounds on isolated human erectile tissue. Eur Urol. 2002 Nov;42(5):523-8

5. Taddei S, Virdis A, Ghiadoni L, Salvetti G, Bernini G, Magagna A, Salvetti A. Age-related reduction of NO availability and oxidative stress in humans. Hypertension. 2001 Aug;38(2):274-9.

6. Guoyao WU, Morris SM. Arginine Metabolism: nitric oxide and beyond. Biochem J 1998; 336:1-17

7. Tomasian D, Keaney JF, Vita JA Antioxidants and the bioactivity of endothelium-derived nitric oxide. Cardiovasc Res. 2000 Aug 18;47(3):426-35.

8. Wollin SD, Jones PJ. Alpha-lipoic acid and cardiovascular disease. J Nutr. 2003 Nov;133(11):3327-30 Guoyao W, Meininger CJ. Arginine Nutrition and Cardiovascular Function. J Nutr.2000;130: 2626-2629

9. Elam RP, et al. Effects of Arginine and Ornithine on Strength, Lean Body Mass and Urinary Hydroxyproline in Adult Males. J Sports Med Phys Fitness. Mar1989;29(1):52-56.

Chapter 16

The "Gold Mind" of Sex

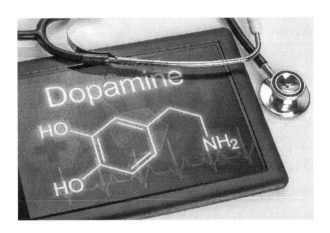

Your body is here with her but your mind is on the other side of town. This scenario is often played out in the more familiar sense as a form of performance anxiety or undesirable brain neurotransmitters. When it comes to having great sex there are at least four essential treasures that every warrior must have in their "Gold Mind." What are they? I call it the holy brain alchemy. They are dopamine, serotonin, prolactin and oxytocin. All of these neural and hormonal compounds are important and necessary for healthy brain sex mood fitness.

What Is Serotonin?

Serotonin is a neurotransmitter that is located in our gastrointestinal tract. What is serotonin? Well, serotonin is a chemical that takes control of our moods, sleep, and appetite, learning ability, concentration level and memory. Eighty percent of the body's serotonin level is produced in the gastrointestinal track. You are what you eat. Serotonin can impact cellular growth, stimulate our metabolism and help with our digestion. It also greatly affects our social behavior and impulses. It is one of the most

important sixteen chemicals in our body. The serotonin present in our gastrointestinal tract gives signals to our brain but when deficient may cause depression and many other problems.

Serotonin is important because it helps to regulate one's mood and can prevent depression. If a man is clinically depressed he probably won't be in the best mood to have sex. In contrast, if one's serotonin levels are too high then there is usually a decline of interest in appetite and sex. Dopamine can also be out of balance and cause too much lust, craving or addiction for sex.

It is my opinion, that a 60-40% brain profile in favor of dopamine to serotonin is probably best for a healthy libido.

The brain is truly the most important sexual organ in the body. Visualization of self being virile, erected and pumped up for vigorous sex is paramount to having good sex. A pornographic mindset sometimes can initially boost some men testosterone levels to the sky. Most men are visually graphic by nature. Romanticism tends to work better for women in general. Sometimes too much attention and focus is placed on the genitals and testosterone while neglecting a healthy gold mind balance.

Albert Einstein once said that "Imagination is more important than knowledge".

Most scientists knew that Einstein often engaged in what is called thought experiments because the technology was not yet developed to prove or test his theories. A sexual warrior too should indulge in thought experiments with a woman of his desire who is more than anxious to please him. Instead of focusing on the woman you want, try focusing your time and energy on the woman that wants you.

"Don't be a man that needs a woman but rather the man that a woman needs".

The brain and the mind set are the commanders and directors who orchestrate our sexual experiences.
Having a good neural conductor can mean the difference between good and bad sex. It is necessary to program the brain to respond and process signals coming from the body to the brain or brain to the body. This is sometimes referred to as neural linguistic programming. We must first understand the nature and nurture of our unique neurotransmitters. Ok, let's start with dopamine.

What is Dopamine?
Dopamine is sometimes referred to as the lust or pleasure hormone. It is a neurotransmitter that helps control the brain's reward and pleasure centers. Dopamine is a neurotransmitter, which is a chemical released by nerve cells to send signals to other nerve cells. Dopamine plays a major role in the brain's biofeedback system that is responsible for reward-driven learning. Every type of reward that has been studied increases the level of dopamine transmission in the brain.

Dopamine improves sexual health causing noticeable increases in arousal, orgasm and mood for both men and women. Dopamine also helps regulate movement and emotional responses. It enables us not only to see rewards, but to take action to move toward them. I simply call it the motivation neurotransmitter. Having a severe dopamine deficiency from a medical standpoint can result in Parkinson's Disease.

People with low dopamine activity may be more prone to addiction. The presence of a certain kind of dopamine receptor is also associated with sensation-seeking. Dopamine is a signaling feedback for predicted rewards such as sexual pleasure. One learns to associate different forms of pleasure with different experiences thus forming a strong connection in the

brain. This connection creates a dopamine link that can be triggered by physical and social cues. We train our own brains to respond in a specific way. The sight of a beautiful women, the release of pheromones or the anticipation of physical pleasure can trigger the release of dopamine.

While dopamine has just five receptor types, another neurotransmitter, serotonin, has 14 currently known sites.

The main biofeedback players are dopamine, the reward elixir, prolactin, the hormone of satiation, oxytocin, the cuddle hormone, and androgen receptors. These 5 key players are all powerful. They can affect our mood, our desire for intimacy, our perception of our mate, as well as our susceptibility to addictive activities and substances.

Sexual orgasm is generally regarded as the ultimate goal of recreational sex. During the course of an orgasm, there is an intense discharge of bio-energy or qi. The result is a cathartic release of excess energy leading to a more relaxed self fulfilled state.
When we are sexually aroused by close contact our dopamine level rises dramatically and at the time of orgasm, we have a dopamine explosion. So how do we know if our dopamine level is in the normal range?

The following chart gives us a general guideline of what is normal to what is excessive.

Excess	Deficient	Normal
Sexual fetishes	Lack of ambition and drive	Healthy libido
Sexual addiction	Inability to "love"	Good feelings toward others
Unhealthy risk-taking	Low libido	Healthy bonding

Low dopamine levels can cause depression, loss of motor control, loss of satisfaction, addictions, cravings, compulsions, low sex drive, poor attention and focus. When dopamine levels are elevated too quickly to a high level, a person may manifest symptoms in the form of anxiety, paranoia, or hyperactivity. Here are some important questions that may reveal the status of one's dopamine level.

Self- Check Questions:

Do you often feel depressed, flat, bored, and apathetic?

Are you low on physical or mental energy?

Do you feel tired a lot and have to push yourself to exercise?

Is your drive, enthusiasm and motivation on the low side?

Do you have difficulty focusing or concentrating?

Are you easily chilled? Do you have cold hands or feet?

Do you tend to put on weight too easily?

Do you feel the need to get more alert and motivated by consuming a lot of coffee or other "uppers" like sugar, diet soda, ephedra, or cocaine?

If you answered yes to 3 or more of the above, then you probably have low dopamine levels. Dopamine levels are depleted by stress, certain antidepressants, drug use, poor nutrition, and poor sleep. Alcohol, caffeine, and sugar all seem to decrease dopamine activity in the brain. Foods that increase dopamine sources by increasing tyrosine include almonds, avocados, bananas, dairy products, lima beans, pumpkin seeds, and sesame seeds.

Dopamine is easily oxidized by the body. Foods that are rich in antioxidants such as fruits and vegetables may help protect dopamine-using neurons from free radical damage.

Many healthcare professionals recommend supplementing with vitamins C, vitamin E, and other antioxidants. Foods such as sugar, excess saturated fats, cholesterol from trans fats, and refined foods interfere
with proper brain function and can cause low
dopamine. Consumption of excess saturated fats and cholesterol should also be reduced because they can clog the arteries to the brain, heart, and other organs in certain individuals.
Caffeine must also be avoided by persons with depression. Caffeine is a stimulant which initially speeds up neurotransmission by temporarily raising the amount of serotonin and elevating one's mood.

Another important source of dopamine are amino acids. Proteins are high in amino acids, which are necessary for dopamine production. They include foods such as fish, eggs, chicken, turkey and red meat to supply your body with adequate amino acids. Fermented soy products such as tempeh and miso and other legumes are considered incomplete proteins; however, they form a more complete protein profile when eaten in combination with grains, becoming excellent sources for dopamine-related amino acids.

Vegetables

Certain vegetables are excellent sources of amino acids that stimulate dopamine production. For example, beets supply the amino acid called betaine, that aids in the regulation of neurotransmitters like dopamine. Artichokes and avocados have also been found to increase dopamine levels.

Fruits

Ripe bananas are a major source of tyrosine. As bananas continue to ripen and become sweeter, their tyrosine component becomes more potent. Tyrosine helps regulate and stimulate dopamine levels, increasing memory and alertness. Apples also are highly recommended for being high in quercetin, a potent antioxidant. Apples can aid in the prevention of neural degenerative diseases by triggering the production of dopamine in the brain. Remember to eat strawberries, blueberries and prunes to round out the best fruit nutrients that trigger dopamine release.

Nuts and Seeds

Raw almonds, sesame and pumpkin seeds make a great snack and help regulate dopamine levels.

Almond butter or tahini, a paste made from sesame seeds, are excellent sources for the amino acids needed for dopamine production.

Wheat Germ

Wheat germ supplies the essential amino acid phenylalanine, that's converted to tyrosine, which then stimulates additional dopamine release. Do not use wheat germ if you are gluten intolerant or allergic to wheat.

Herbs

Several common herbs are known for helping to regulate dopamine levels. These include stinging nettle, fenugreek, ginseng, milk thistle, red clover, and peppermint. They are best consumed as herbal teas.

Vitamin Supplements

Adding supplements to your diet to increase dopamine levels may be helpful if you're unable to get those nutrients from foods. Tyrosine, plus several vitamins such as B, C and E as well as iron, folic acid and niacin all help to trigger dopamine release.

Check with your health care practitioner before including additional iron in your diet.

Following sexual orgasm, men's dopamine level tends to decrease sharply and can be described as a form of "Post-Orgasm Hangover." This reaction is however delayed in women. Men can also expect prolactin levels to rise, and androgen receptors to fall after an orgasm. These disruptive high-low neural hormonal chemical cycles of orgasm can cause a bit of confusion for those searching for a stable sex life.

Serotonin and endorphin levels usually rise after an orgasm while dopamine levels decrease. In other words, when serotonin levels increase dopamine levels tend to decrease. Simply put, if you are feeling too happy then you probably don't crave sex or need it. When it comes to sex a little bit of tension is good.

For those of you who are disciplined enough to practice tantra or the Taoist Seminal Retention Method, dopamine (lust, craving and motivation) levels can be maintained at higher levels for longer periods postponing satiation.
  The practice of tantra sexual union offers a viable solution to the disruptive high-low neural chemical cycles of orgasm.

Women on the other hand have a distinct advantage over men in their ability to have multiple orgasms while maintaining adequate dopamine levels with a postponing of prolactin.

Men on the other, tend to trade off control for one peak explosive orgasm that usually lead to fatigue. This drop from sustained dopamine levels or desire usually results in the need for sleep or a recovery period of several days, quite similar to that of weight training. One of the primary goal of the sexual warrior should be to increase sexual potential by delaying prolactin and maintaining adequate dopamine levels during a sexual encounter. Both partners can now enjoy foreplay and after play with minimum depletion of energy reserve. The male does not have to make a sacrifice of his sexual energy just to have an orgasm.

The sexual warrior should always be prepared to satisfy himself as well as his lover. He should look forward with confidence that each future sexual encounter will be as enjoyable and intense as the last. The tantra method offers a win/win scenario for both partners. It is well worth the time and discipline to learn and master.

Sex is best understood in the context of bio-energy or life-force, also called prana, chi (qi), ki, orgone or mana. All living objects possess an outer and innermost aura that can be sensed or seen by certain sensitive individuals. Many experience this energy as a form of heat or tingling sensation in the body. The sex chakra is our strongest bio-energy generator. This energy center provides a moderate stream of energy into the base chakra and then up the spine into the brain, it also maintains the production of our sex hormones. If this energy generator becomes weak, we could easily lose our vitality and become
more susceptible to premature aging and disease.

It is important that we don't over or under utilize our sexual energy generator or chakra. The sexual warrior should never forget that frequent ejaculation tends to deplete our energy. Too much abstinence from sex on the other hand can be just as bad by snuffing out our inner fire. The logical solution would be to make sufficient use or stimulation of our sexual energy without over depleting our vital essence. This energy should be ultimately channeled into the chakra and acupuncture system to keep us young and healthy.

Sexual energy must be channeled upward to the brain and back to body for both physical and mental rejuvenation. Over stimulation of the brain can lead to imbalances and insanity. Mantak Chia's book on "Cultivating Male Sexual Energy", emphasized the practice of the microcosmic circulation of energy method.

This method is meditative in nature and helps to establish and maintain the correct mind and body harmony to balance the flow of energy(qi). When using this method, energy or qi is circulated in a balanced way from the base sex chakra to the brain and back to the body continuously during sexual intercourse.

Now let's talk about frequency of intercourse. If you can recall earlier in this book, I mentioned something about the Taoist schedule for seminal ejaculation. This schedule is based upon a man's age, vitality and desire. A mathematical formula was deduced by the Taoists based upon careful observation and long-term research.

This secret formula is derived by multiplying a man's age by 0.2, for example, a 20-year-old x 0.2 = 4.4 days of recovery needed to achieve a full charge of vitality for the next encounter. On the other hand, a 60-year-old man x 0.2 can require 12 days minimum to recharge after an intense encounter.

Frequency of Sex:
Frequency of sex usually depends on the desire and health of a couple. On a shorter time scale, a 30 minute intercourse period is adequate for most couples in general with a five day interval. If a sexual encounter endures for one hour then the need for future intercourse would be more or less on a 7-day schedule. If a couple is healthy enough to have sex for up to two hours then a two-week interval would seen like the norm. Again, it all depends upon if the couple is healthy and robust enough to have sex for such an extended period.

 In any case, taking a sufficient break according to one's age and vitality is important in order to fully recharge the bodies battery with bio-energy or qi for future encounters. Keep in mind, its quality that out rates quantity.

References:

University of Maryland Medical Center: Tyrosine
University of Michigan Health System: L-Tyrosine
Middle Tennessee State University: Food, Mood and Neurotransmitters
James Madison University: How Dopamine is Made in the Brain

Tyrosine Benefits
MedHelp.com

Chapter 17

Exercise and Sexual Fitness

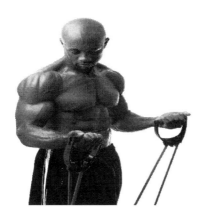

In this chapter, we will explore the many aspects of exercises that impact the functioning of the male reproductive system. Good sex is a good thing.

Though definitions vary, "good sex" might be thought of as an act of intimacy that promotes health, pleasure and well-being. Good sex provides significant physical and psychological benefits.

Let us revisit the number one question discussed previously in this book.

Are you healthy enough to have great sex?

Explore the following questions:

Do you have low back pain?

Can you run up a flight of stairs without collapsing?

Do I have good stamina and endurance to do physical labor?

Are you over-weight?

Are you experiencing adrenal burnout from chronic stress?

Do you sleep 6-8 hours of sleep per night?

Are you emotionally or mentally balanced?

Do you have frequent urination at night?

If the answers to several of these questions are yes, be realistic and take action to improve your core health. Placing demands on yourself to be a stallion in the bedroom may not be a reality based option. The good news is that research shows there is a reciprocal relationship between one's health and sexual readiness. Solving the physical problems can often remedy the sexual issues as well.

General Guideline Summary

- Increase muscle mass and decrease body fat levels

-Increase intake of vitamin D3, C, B, calcium and magnesium combined at a 2:1 ratio.

-Avoid junk denatured or processed foods

-Eat according to the testosterone diet plan outlined in my previous chapter.

-Monitor and decrease your exposure to xenoestrogen chemicals.

-Practice orgasm without ejaculation periodically or postponing it to enhance sex drive, and maintain adequate dopamine levels which usually diminish after intercourse. This method is sometimes referred to as edging or seminal retention.

-Be aware that regular exposure to pornography can raise or lower dopamine levels and thus require one to need even higher levels of visual stimulation. I call it the negative porno feedback loop. Leave some excitement to your own imagination.

-Avoid intense stimulus found in internet porn and other graphic sexual content. Reducing the need or obsession for hardcore porn should be part of your sexual mind de-conditioning program.

-Over stimulation is just as bad as under-stimulation.

Now, what are the best exercises to enhance one's sexual potential? Well, the best exercises should all share common attributes.

These common attributes are increased oxygen, blood circulation, the release of free testosterone, nitric oxide, HGH, raising dopamine

levels, pelvic strength, endurance, mental focus and improve energy or qi. In order to achieve these results, the following topics will be reviewed starting with Muscle Resistance Training.

Muscle Resistance Training

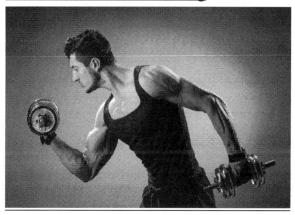

Many experts advocate the slow control lifting of weights or doing short reps with a heavy weight to stimulate the body's testosterone level. The goal here is intensity not endurance.

In fact, some studies have linked short intense exercise such as weight lifting with increased testosterone levels. Lighter weights with higher repetition can also be advantageous by increasing definition and lean body tissue thus creating more receptor cells site for testosterone.

In order to improve your sex life, do some push-ups, sit-ups, and crunches at least 3 times a week.

These muscle-building exercises can help lead to better sex by strengthening the shoulders, chest, and abs. Strong upper body strength can increase stamina since these muscles are used during intercourse.

Cold and Hunger

When we are feeling cold from the weather or artificially induced cold such as a cold bath or shower our bodies often respond by revving up testosterone levels dramatically for survival reasons. One of my most esteemed friends, mentor and martial arts teacher Raymond, moved to Sweden for this very reason. Every morning around 5 am, he goes outdoors virtually nude and exposes himself to frigid temperatures. Please do not try this without proper training and supervision. The monks in Tibet refer to this austere form of training and meditation as

Tum-Mo Yoga. Tibetan monks have demonstrated under rigorous scientific scrutiny the ability to raise their core body temperatures in a freezing environment and endure cold beyond the limits of most people.

Raymond has adopted this form of cold training in an effort to heal and regenerate his body of old war injuries. Many of his injuries were the result of agent orange herbicide exposure and rocket shrapnel while on assignment in Vietnam. At the age of 72, Raymond is remarkably healthy, youthful, robust and fit. He attributes his gains to cryogenic therapy or Tibetan Tum-Mo.

Cold weather often can trigger hunger in the body causing us to consume more calories. When the urge to eat and stay warm is postponed for a reasonably amount of time, our bodies will reward us by triggering a surge release of testosterone and HGH. The combination of both cold and intermittent fasting is a wonderful way to boost hormones safely and increase one's longevity. If you live in a warm tropical environment try standing under a waterfall or swimming in a cold spring. While visiting Florida during the summer, I would often swim in cold springs such as Ginnie Springs and Devil's Grotto. After swimming in the water for about 5-10 minutes I would feel a noticeable testosterone surge.

Kegels

Men can use the Kegel method to delay ejaculation by contracting their inner genital anal muscles just before orgasm. Kegel exercises can be done by interrupting the flow of urine when going to the bathroom. This will help to become better acquainted with your PC muscles. The good news is that you can do Kegels anytime and any place by squeezing the PC muscles. Hold for 10 seconds, relax, and do as many reps as you can before tiring.

Kegels are considered to be a good sex exercise for men because these exercises can improve sexual endurance and ejaculation control by toning the pubococcygeus (PC) muscles. These internal muscles allow you stop the flow of urine mid-stream and control premature ejaculation.

Named after the Los Angeles physician Arnold Kegel, this form of training strengthens the muscles in your body's pelvic floor which can lead to better sex.

Speed Walking

In a study of 31,000 men over age 50, Harvard researchers found that aerobic exercise resulted in a 30-percent lower risk of erectile dysfunction. According to another study, aerobic activity that burns at least 200 calories per day (equal to fast walking for two miles) can significantly lower the risk of ED.

Brisk Walking is thought to help ED by improving circulation and blood flow. Fast walking, sprinting, and other exercises activities help your sex life for the same reason that they prevent heart attacks. Aerobic and anaerobic exercises both keep blood vessels clear and flowing.

New research in sport medicine shows that cardio type of exercises done at a set pace should not be performed longer than 20 minutes. These type of exercises can trigger the release of cortisol or stress hormone that tends to lower testosterone. I personally use cardio as a general warmup prior to my high intensity exercises. The result is often stronger and longer erections. These exercises can boost sexual performance when you need it the most.

Swimming

A Harvard study of 160 male and female swimmers in their 60s reported sex lives comparable to those in their 40s. Since sexual activity can be an act of endurance, long-distance swimming can keep you going and going like the energizer bunny. Swimming for at least 30 minutes three times a week will increase sexual endurance when you need it the most. The colder the water the more intense the effect it has on testosterone. Cold water baths and showers can also increase the production of testosterone

Vigorous Dirty Dancing (VDG)

Dancing in a sexually provocative manner can raise the bar on one's libido and dopamine levels serving as a warm up to sex. Dirty Dancing done right can easily activate the core, hip, butt and rotational muscles that are heavily engaged when having good sex. Try dancing at least 15-20 minutes or 3-5 songs in a row. Try not to over do it but build up your intensity gradually. VDG will activate and strengthen the gluteal muscles (the gluteus maximus, medius and minimus) making them stronger and better toned.

Not only can you improve the appearance of your backside, you can also improve your sex life. These muscles help support, rotate and extend your trunk and hips. This means that during intercourse, they contribute to thrusting action.

Pelvic Bridges

Pelvic bridges give you a bonus of core strength and flexibility of the lower back. Lie on your back with knees bent, feet flat on the floor shoulder-width apart. Raise your pelvic region in a straight line like a bridge. Hold your abdominals in while you tighten your glutes and push your inner thighs toward each other. Slowly lower to the floor and repeat, 20 to 25 reps.

Yoga

Benefits of yoga exercises for male sexual health have been well documented in the system of ayurvedic medicine from India. Yoga benefits:

Helps raises the vibration of sexual energy, so it can be used for healing and spiritual transformation.

Helps develop sexual potency and improves sex drive.

Helps cure sexual dysfunction and sexual phobias.

Helps cure erectile dysfunction. Yoga increases energy and vitality in general. Significantly develops lower body strength and flexibility. It tones legs and buttocks awakens, heals and balances the Sex Chakra.

The Plank

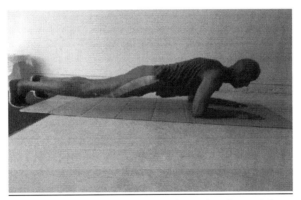

Dr. Isom performing the Plank Bridge

There is one move that can make you more sexually confident, daring and strong?

It is called the plank. The plank is a core-building exercise popular in yoga and martial arts. This type of exercise works multiple muscle groups simultaneously such as the upper arms, abdominals, obliques, thighs and buttocks. These important muscles groups help to stabilize you when engaged in intercourse on all fours, any mounted top positions or other positional changes.

Lay face down with the palms of your hands flat on the floor on each side of your shoulders. In this position, your forearms should also be flat on the floor and used as a fulcrum support to raise your body. Push your weight to the balls of your feet as you push up onto your forearms and palms. Your entire body should now be suspended in the air.

Be careful to keep your body as straight and flat as possible and avoid lifting your butt in the air. Hold this position for 10 seconds then relax for a few seconds before repeating. Work up to one minute.

Yoga Cobra Poise

Cobra Pose can be used to help balance and heal the sex chakra according to ayurvedic medicine. This posture directs nerve current and blood flow to the genital areas. It is well worth mastering. If your arms get tired, come down from cobra and then go back into the pose after recovering.

Duration: 30 seconds – 3 minutes.

Breath Pattern: Long deep rhythmic breathing.

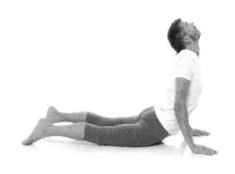

The Plough

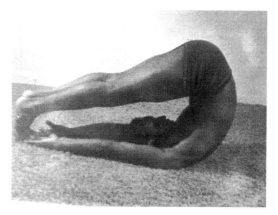

Dr. Isom in the plough position

As a mindful precaution, please develop your capacity to do the plough pose slowly and gently. Be careful with your neck and do not over strain. The position shown above is an advanced posture. Improving the flexibility in your hamstrings will help you with doing this pose as well. This pose is an excellent asana or posture to improve your back and reproductive systems.

Duration: 1 – 3 minutes

Breath: long deep breathing.

plough pose is used for sexual healing

Please develop your capacity to do this pose slowly and gently. Be careful with your back. There are also modified versions of the plough.

For more information visit

http://www.yogaoutlet.com/guides/how-to-do-plow-pose-in-yoga

The Yoga Chair Poise for Sex

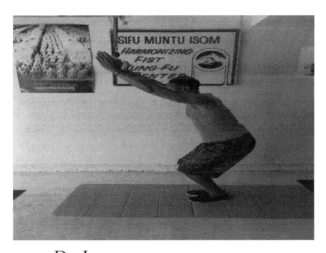

Dr. Isom

We now get to the exercises which really start to work the lower body and legs. This exercise can be another source of sexual power and energy. Be careful with your knees.

Remember, you can take breaks in between if you need to. The chair pose is both a posture and stance quite common to many forms of internal martial arts such as Tai Ji, Xing–I and Bagua.

Breath of Fire

Do a series of rhythmic bellow like breathing with emphasis on your abdominal muscle groups. This type of breathing can generate lots of internal heat in your body. Drink ample amounts of water when you are done. Breathe in and out rapidly while bellowing your abdominal muscles repeatedly.
Duration: 15 seconds – 3 minutes

Internal Martial Arts

This form of martial arts includes arts such as Tai Ji, Bagua Zhang and Xing-I Chuan. Internal martial arts tend to focus more on relaxation, meditation in motion with an emphasis on health and longevity. In contrast, external forms of martial arts like kick boxing or karate tend stress the over-development of external muscles, dynamic tension and fighting.

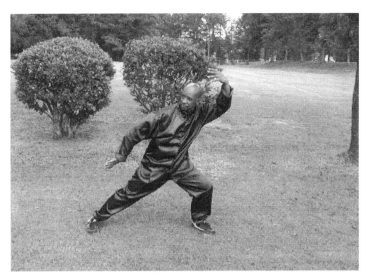
Dr. Isom, The Bagua Celestial Stem Posture

Internal exercises such as Bagua Zhang emphasizes the development of both the spiral and circular energy. Martial arts students can build a good foundation in this art by walking the circle and practicing both forms and application.

Qigong

Another great physical discipline and art to raise one's sexual energy through the roof is qigong. This art emphasizes the cultivation of qi through deep breathing, balanced postures and meditation. It only takes a few minutes a day to keep the libido strong. There are 400 different forms of Qigong. If you are interested see my book and video on Life Is Healing Medical Qigong at www.lifeishealing.com

Qigong exercises and proper diet can help a man to maintain his sexual performance without the use of drugs and male hormone therapy.

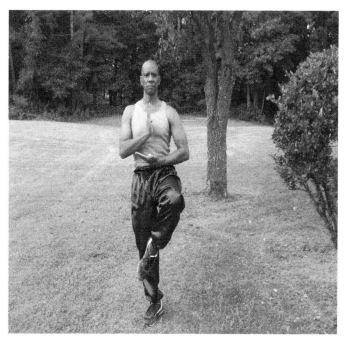

Dr. Isom
Buddha Standing on the Post

Qigong is easy to learn but difficult to master. In the future, I hope to be able to create a manual of therapeutic sexual exercises specifically designed to address male sexual energy.

Visit my website for future updates, products and services. Phone/Skype consults are available by appointment. For more info go to

www.lifeishealing.com

www.harmonizingfist.com

References:

http://thepenisadvantage.com

Article Source:

http://EzineArticles.com/?expert=Nick_Stevens

Article Source: http://EzineArticles.com/3710029

Mayo Clinic Staff. Men's Health: preventing your top 10 risks. MayoClinic.org.

http://www.mayoclinic.com/health/mens-health/MC00013. Accessed Dec. 22, 2009.

Staying Healthy after 40. AOLHealth.com.

http://www.aolhealth.com/health/mens-health/advice-for-men-over-40. Accessed Dec. 22, 2009.

Stretching Exercises. Men's Health.

http://www.menshealth.com/men/fitness/muscle-building/stretching-exercises/article/472a99edbbbd201099edbbbd2010cfe793cd. Accessed Dec. 22, 2009.

Zamora. D. Men's Top 5 Health Concerns.

WebMD.com. http://men.webmd.com/features/mens-top-5-health-concerns. Accessed Dec. 22, 2009.

Bonus Chapter 18

What is Hypogonadism?

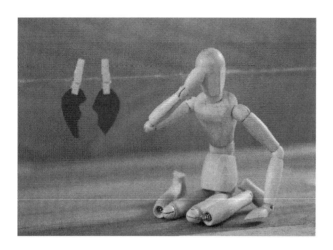

Hypogonadism is a medical glandular disorder. This medical condition is one of the major causes of low testosterone level in men and low estrogen in women. A common colloquial expression for this condition describes it as a case of "Broken Balls."

- Primary Hypogonadism (Pituitary gland functions normally but the testes are not getting the signal to respond appropriately. The Leydig Cells in the testes are damaged or atrophied. (T levels <200)
- Secondary Hypogonadism The pituitary gland does not function well in producing LH/FSH. The testes do not get the signal to make testosterone.
- Tertiary Hypogonadism The hypothalamus does not secrete enough GnRH for the pituitary gland to make LH/FSH.

- Luteinizing Stimulating Hormone (LSH) makes testosterone.
- Follicle Stimulating Hormone (FSH) makes sperm
- Conventional Treatment is Bio-Identical Hormone or Hormone Replacement Therapy (HRT) or (TRT).

What are the causes of Hypogonadism?

Some of the more common causes are as follows:

1. Prolonged use of anabolic steroid cause the testes and penis to shrinks due to the negative feedback loop of endogenous testosterone.

2. Aid/HIV induced hypogonadism causing glandular dysfunction causing low levels of testosterone to impact the hypothalamus, pituitary and testes.

3. Prolonged celibacy and a sedentary monastic lifestyle.

4. Certain diseases can contribute to hypogonadism such as Diabetes Type 2 leading to metabolic syndrome, inflammatory diseases, tuberculosis and sarcoidosis.

5. Failure of the testicles to descend during puberty causing developmental delays. If not corrected in early childhood, it may lead to malfunction of the testicles and reduced production of testosterone.

6. Neutering/castration of a male by removing the testes.

7. Medications and the use of certain drugs like opiate pain killers can affect testosterone production

8. Obesity being significantly overweight at any age may be linked to hypogonadism.

9. Normal aging can render older men in general to lower testosterone levels than younger men. As men age, there's a slow and continuous decrease in testosterone production.

10. Chronic stress can cause the reproductive system can temporarily shut down due to the physical stress of an illness or surgery, as well as during significant emotional stress. This is a result of diminished signals from the hypothalamus and usually resolves with successful treatment of the underlying condition.

There are many symptoms associated with hypogonadism. These symptoms may occur early in life, during puberty or into adulthood.

Puberty

Male hypogonadism may delay puberty or cause incomplete or lack of normal development. It can cause:

Decreased development of muscle mass

- Lack of deepening of the voice
- Impaired growth of body hair
- Impaired growth of the penis and testicles

- Excessive growth of the arms and legs in relation to the trunk of the body
- Development of breast tissue (gynecomastia)

Adulthood

In adult males, hypogonadism may alter certain masculine physical characteristics and impair normal reproductive function. Signs and symptoms may include:

- Erectile dysfunction
- Infertility
- Decrease in beard and body hair growth
- Decrease in muscle mass
- Development of breast tissue (gynecomastia)
- Loss of bone mass (osteoporosis)

Hypogonadism can also cause mental and emotional changes. As testosterone decreases, some men may experience symptoms similar to those of menopause in women. These may include:

- Fatigue
- Decreased sex drive
- Difficulty concentrating
- Hot flashes

Conventional Medical Treatment doses not seek a cure but is geared toward management using endogenous testosterone gels, injected subcutaneous pellets and testosterone injections. The more common mode of treatment is the used for hypogonadism is a hormone called (HCG) Human Chorionic Gonadotropin.

- Intramuscular injections are the most cost-effective form. Injections are given every two weeks. Often produces fluctuations in hormone levels and recurrence of symptoms between doses.
- Transdermal patches are the closest to normal hormone production. They need to be applied to the skin each night. Local skin irritation may occur.
- Transdermal gels 1% testosterone gel. Applied once a day. Can be transferred to others, partner or to children, through contact.
- Nasal testosterone gel recently approved in the United States. This may resolve the issue of person to person transfer.

Holistic treatment option emphasizes prevention healthy lifestyle, proper diet, exercises, restoring and maintaining a healthy endocrine balance using supplementation and herbal formulations. Maintaining a lean muscle mass and reducing fat or estrogen receptors while increasing androgen receptor cell sites can lead to a cure and long-term solution.

It is important for a warrior to understand the purpose and function of The Hypothalamus Pituitary Gonad Axis. This axis is the basis for understanding the how and why men suffer from hypogonadism and how to treat it.

THE HYPOTHALMUS PITUITARY GONAD AXIS (HPGA)
(Simplified)

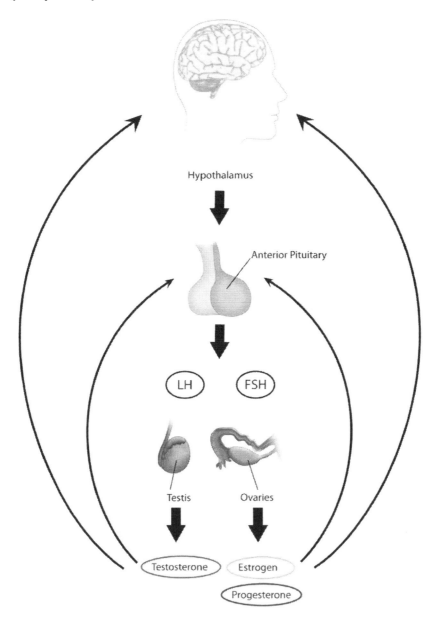

Nitric Oxide Killer Enzyme

Another killer enzyme is called phosphodiesterase type 5 or PDE-5. The PDE-5 enzyme neutralizes a bodily compound called guanosine monophosphate or (cGMP). The cGMP compound is responsible for triggering the release of nitric oxide which is a naturally occurring vasodilator.

If you recalled, vasodilators are necessary to engorge the penis with blood so that a healthy firm erection can be achieved. As cGMP increases, the smooth muscles of the penile arteries relax allowing the vessels to dilate and increase blood flow to the penis. Remember, cGMP is one of our best allies in the war against erection killers and must be protected.

What else does a sexual warrior needs to know know?

Every warrior needs to know about sex pills that don't really live up to their claims and comes with a price on health. The first and most marketed pill sold worldwide is Viagra. What is Viagra? It is known as a PDE-5 Inhibitor. Let's know explore them and their shortcomings.

PDE-5 Inhibitor Viagra/Levitra Design Flaw

There are inherent design flaws that present in the development of Viagra type drugs.

Viagra was originally design for to be used as heart medication to allow for greater blood flow through the coronary arteries and other blood vessels. Many past heart patients began noticing the unexpected positive side effect of increase erections while taking this medicine.

Shortly after, many pharmaceutical companies began exploiting this side effect and marketing the drug as a blue sex wonder pill. It is important to under benefit risk factors when taking any new drug. Viagra is not a perfect long-term solution for increasing male sexual performance. Here are some of the limitations of Viagra and other similar drugs.

- Without proper blood flow to the clitoris, women cannot have orgasms or experience enhanced sexual sensitivity neither can men.
- PDE5 Inhibitors like Viagra was not designed as a long -term solution.
- They are ineffective in many people whose NO levels are too low from the start.
- Their effect diminishes over time. They become ineffective for 50% of all user after
- 3 years.

Viagra Side Effects (Sildenafil Citrate) PDE-5 Inhibitor allows cGMP to activate NO2(Caveat > Does not work without proper arousal.)

Common Side Undesirable Effects:

- Aches or pains in the muscles
- bloody nose
- diarrhea
- difficult or labored breathing
- Sexual activity may put extra strain on your heart
- headache
- pain or tenderness around the eyes and cheekbones
- redness of the skin
- sneezing
- stomach discomfort following meals
- stuffy or runny nose
- trouble sleeping
- unusually warm skin
- Vision Changes increased sensitivity to light, blurred vision
- Trouble discriminating blue and green colors

A sexual warrior must also be knowledgeable of what is called the luteinizing hormonal process.

Luteinizing hormone, (LH) is a hormone that helps regulate reproductive processes in males and females. It is produced by the pituitary gland. In women, luteinizing hormones helps regulate the menstrual cycle and ovulation. In men, this hormone stimulates the production of testosterone in the testicles, which plays an important role in producing sperm. Determining the amount of luteinizing hormones present is a common step in investigating infertility in women and men.

If the LH level is high during a urine or blood test, indications are positive for a low testosterone production. Abnormally high levels of the hormone in men may indicate that the testicles are not functioning or have been removed.

Afterword

The paradigm of sexual health in the future will be based on mind, body, energy flow integration rather than the mere use of pharmaceuticals, hormone replacement or steroidal compounds. The Sexual Warrior Within addresses the fine points of male sexual health utilizing safe non- invasive modalities. Eastern and western herbal compounds, cycling with seasonal rotation, testosterone diet and Chinese energetic sexual tantra practices are some of the practices presented in this book.

Many of the sexual esoteric guarded secrets about sex were kept away from the mainstream population and privileged to only a few. The Sexual Warrior Within captures both theory and practice while offering a multitude of alternative approaches and solutions.

Sexual issues such as impotence, low libido, erectile dysfunction etc. are fully explored in detail. The Sexual Warrior Within encompasses the physics of male sexuality in addition to presenting a complete examination of the more compelling sexual issues that need to be addressed.

In conclusion to this book, my final words of encouragement are, Protect, guard and empower the sexual warrior within. "Have a wonderful enduring sex life for both you and your love one."

Dr. Angelo Isom ND/CHS.

The essential information contained in the content of this book can easily be understood and applied by the layman and may be applicable to other professionals canvassing for new ideas and solutions.

Dr. Angelo Isom N.D. CHS, MQT, author, male holistic adviser, researcher, healer, qigong master, martial arts lineage holder and director of Life is Healing Institute.

Made in the USA
Columbia, SC
13 February 2018